SUPER EASY ANTI-INFLAMMATORY DIET FOR BEGINNERS

Discover Quick and Tasty Recipes to Improve Digestion, Boost Your Immune System, And Reduce Stress in Just A Few Weeks. Full Color Edition

Daniel Viona

© **Copyright 2024 by Daniel Viona - All rights reserved.**

The content of this book is provided with the intent to offer accurate and reliable information. However, by purchasing this book, you acknowledge that neither the publisher nor the author claim expertise in the topics discussed, and any advice or recommendations are provided solely for entertainment purposes. It is recommended that you consult with professionals as necessary before taking any action based on the content of this book.

This disclaimer is recognized as fair and valid by both the American Bar Association and the Committee of Publishers Association, and is legally binding across the United States.

Unauthorized transmission, duplication, or reproduction of any part of this work, whether electronic or printed, including the creation of secondary or tertiary copies, or recorded versions, is prohibited without the express written consent of the publisher. All rights not expressly granted are reserved.

The information presented in this book is deemed to be truthful and accurate. However, any negligence in the use or misuse of this information by the reader is their sole responsibility, and under no circumstances will the publisher or the author be liable for any consequences or damages that may arise from the use of this information.

Furthermore, the information contained in this book is intended solely for informational purposes and should be treated as such. No guarantees are made regarding the ongoing validity or quality of the information. Trademarks mentioned are used without permission and their inclusion does not constitute an endorsement by the trademark holder.

TABLE OF CONTENTS

INTRODUCTION 9
1. The Impact of Inflammation 9

CHAPTER 1: UNDERSTANDING INFLAMMATION 13
1. What Is Inflammation? Causes and Triggers 13
2. Symptoms and Health Risks 15

CHAPTER 2: FOOD LIST 19
1. Foods That Fuel Inflammation 19
2. Anti-Inflammatory Foods 21

CHAPTER 3: ESSENTIAL NUTRIENTS FOR REDUCING INFLAMMATION 23
1. Vitamins and Minerals 23
2. Omega-3 Fatty Acids 25
3. Antioxidants and Phytochemicals 27

CHAPTER 6: BREAKFAST RECIPES 31
Golden Turmeric Morning Elixir 31
Green Detox Power Smoothie 32
Blueberry Avocado Bliss Smoothie 32
Spiced Berry Metabolism Booster 33
Pineapple Ginger Immune Booster 33
Turmeric Ginger Chia Pudding 34
Omega Booster Smoothie Bowl 35
Savory Quinoa Breakfast Bowl 35
Berry Antioxidant Oatmeal 36
Sweet Potato & Kale Hash 36

CHAPTER 7: LUNCH RECIPES 38
Kale and Quinoa Power Bowl 38
Chickpea and Avocado Garden Salad 39
Spinach and Strawberry Crisp Salad 40
Roasted Beet and Arugula Salad 40
Mediterranean Lentil Bowl 41
Coconut Curry Soup 41
Grilled Chicken Wrap 42
Hummus and Veggie Sandwich 43
Avocado Chickpea Wrap 43
Turkey and Spinach Sandwich 44

Chapter 8: Dinner Recipes 45

- Herb-Marinated Grilled Salmon 46
- Lemon Garlic Chicken Breasts 46
- Spiced Tofu Stir-Fry 47
- Ginger-Lime Shrimp 47
- Balsamic Glazed Pork Chops 48
- Roasted Cauliflower Steaks with Turmeric and Garlic 49
- Zucchini Noodles with Avocado Pesto 49
- Cauliflower Mac and Cheese 50
- Lentil Bolognese 51
- Chicken and Veggie Casserole 51

Chapter 9: Snacks and Small Bites 53

- Beetroot and Apple Juice 53
- Carrot Ginger Smoothie 54
- Green Apple Kale Juice 54
- Pineapple Turmeric Juice 55
- Berry Antioxidant Smoothie 56
- Almond Coconut Energy Balls 56
- Turmeric Cashew Bites 57
- Date and Walnut Bars 57
- Chia Seed Energy Bites 58
- Pumpkin Spice Protein Balls 59

Chapter 10: Desserts and Treats 60

- Mango Coconut Sorbet 60
- Baked Cinnamon Apples 61
- Grilled Peaches with Honey 61
- Strawberry Basil Salad 62
- Blueberry Chia Pudding 62
- Carrot and Walnut Muffins 63
- Oatmeal Raisin Cookies 64
- Lemon Poppy Seed Scones 64
- Cashew Lime Dream Bites 65
- Avocado Chocolate Mousse 66

Chapter 11: Beverages and Teas 67

- Turmeric Ginger Tea 67
- Chamomile and Lavender Tea 68
- Peppermint and Licorice Root Tea 68
- Hibiscus and Rosehip Tea 69
- Lemon Balm and Ginger Infusion 69
- Golden Milk Smoothie 70

Green Matcha Smoothie 70
Blueberry Spinach Smoothie 71
Ginger Beet Smoothie 71
Pineapple Kale Smoothie 72

CHAPTER 12: CONCLUSION 73
30 DAYS MEAL PLAN 75

INTRODUCTION

Welcome to a journey that may very well transform your life. It's no secret that what we eat significantly impacts our health, but the role of diet in controlling inflammation often goes unnoticed in our busy daily lives. Inflammation, sometimes called a silent fire within, affects countless people, contributing to a host of health issues—from persistent fatigue and digestion problems to more serious conditions like heart disease and diabetes.

Understanding and managing this hidden ailment can seem daunting, especially amidst the noise of countless quick fixes and fad diets that promise much but deliver little. That's where the incredible potential of the anti-inflammatory diet comes into play, and why I felt compelled to write this book. It's more than just about eating; it's about nurturing your body back to health and vitality without feeling overwhelmed.

My mission is to simplify what it means to eat anti-inflammatorily. This book isn't just a collection of recipes—it's a friendly guide, packed with clear explanations, vibrant photos, and practical advice, all laid out to lead you through the ins and outs of reducing inflammation through your diet. Whether you're looking to ease existing health concerns or just improve your overall well-being, you'll find that making small adjustments to your eating habits can have profound effects.

In the following pages, we'll explore what inflammation really is, how it affects your body, and most importantly, the myriad ways you can deliciously eat to dampen its effects. Expect to uncover the myths and understand the facts with ease. We'll go through essential nutrients, straight-to-the-point food lists, and simple, tasty recipes designed to make your journey not only successful but also enjoyable.

Embrace this adventure with an open heart and a willing palate, and let's take these stepping stones to better health together. With each page, you'll be one step closer to feeling energetic, healthier, and yes, even happier. Let's begin.

1. THE IMPACT OF INFLAMMATION

Imagine your body as a highly sophisticated alarm system. When everything is functioning correctly, it safeguards you against real threats—bacteria, viruses, toxins. But sometimes, this system errs by signaling a false alarm, causing your defenses to overreact. This analogy can help you understand the essence of inflammation—a natural process meant to protect and heal yet capable of causing significant harm when it goes awry.

Inflammation in its rightful context is beneficial, a crucial component of your immune system's response to injury or infection. Picture the last time you nicked your finger; the redness, warmth, swelling, and pain were all signs of your immune system at work, fighting off potential infection and mending damaged tissue.

However, the real concern arises when inflammation becomes chronic. Unlike the acute, localized inflammation of a cut, chronic inflammation is a silent and pervasive fire that spreads throughout your body, often without obvious symptoms. This inflammatory response can be triggered by numerous factors, including stress, lifestyle choices, environmental toxins, and most notably, diet. Chronic inflammation has been linked to numerous health issues, some of which affect millions globally. Diseases such as arthritis, heart disease, diabetes, and even neurological conditions like Alzheimer's can all have a root in sustained inflammatory responses. This makes understanding and managing inflammation through lifestyle choices—notably diet—an essential strategy for long-term health.

Given its stealthy nature, many people live with chronic inflammation without even realizing it until more serious health issues arise. Common signs include continuous fatigue, digestive problems, and in some cases, vague aches and pains that defy clear diagnosis. Identifying these symptoms early can be the key to curtailing their impact, opening a pathway to targeted dietary strategies to quell this underlying inflammation.

The link between diet and inflammation is both profound and empowering. Foods act as signals in our bodies, and certain types can trigger inflammatory responses. For example, processed sugars and trans fats are known culprits that can stimulate inflammation. Conversely, there are foods rich in antioxidants, omega-3 fatty acids, and phytochemicals known to fight inflammation. The power to tilt the balance of your body's inflammatory state is largely in your hands, or more aptly, on your plate.

One of the most compelling pieces of research in nutritional science has been the observation of populations who subsist on traditional Mediterranean or Okinawan diets—both of which are rich in anti-inflammatory components like fish, nuts, leafy greens, and healthy oils. These populations tend to have lower incidences of chronic diseases and longer life expectancies.

The underlying mechanism revolves around how certain foods influence the molecular pathways that activate inflammation. For instance, omega-3 fatty acids—abundant in fish like salmon and sardines—help produce resolvins, which are powerful anti-inflammatory compounds. Meanwhile, colorful fruits and vegetables are loaded with antioxidants that reduce oxidative stress, a key promoter of inflammation.

Understanding this, the question arises: How can this knowledge be packaged into practical, daily eating habits without making meal preparation a daunting task? This is where the beauty of simplicity comes in—I advocate for a straightforward approach to incorporating anti-inflammatory foods in your diet. Small, consistent changes, like adding a serving of leafy greens to each meal or swapping refined grains for whole ones, can lead to significant impacts over time. Much more than a trend, an anti-inflammatory diet is a return to the basics of eating—choosing whole, unprocessed foods. This practice isn't merely about reducing inflammation; it's about nourishing your body in a way that naturally minimizes the risk of disease. It's a lifestyle aimed at celebrating a diverse array of foods that not only taste good but also inherently provide the nutrients necessary to calm inflammatory processes.

The battle against chronic inflammation is a testament to the classic adage that prevention is better than cure. By understanding the impact of inflammation and the role our diet plays, we're equipped not just to live, but to thrive. The commitment to an anti-inflammatory diet is a step towards reclaiming control of your health, providing a firm foundation on which all else can flourish.

In essence, think of managing inflammation as tending a garden: it requires regular attention and care. With the right tools—knowledge of which foods heal and which harm—you can cultivate a state of health that allows your body, your personal landscape, to thrive. This journey you're about to embark on is not about following a restrictive diet; it's about learning to make choices that harmonize with your body's inherent needs. As you turn the page, remember that each step forward is a step towards a more vibrant, healthier you.

Chapter 1: Understanding Inflammation

Welcome to a transformative journey through the understanding of inflammation: your body's silent alarm signal. When it comes to protecting itself against injuries or infections, our body's immune system brilliantly kicks into gear. However, imagine this reaction happening constantly, even when there's no apparent danger. This is where the tale of chronic inflammation begins, quietly shaping many of our most daunting health challenges.

Inflammation is not inherently villainous. In its acute form, characterized by the heat, pain, redness, and swelling that follows a stubbed toe or a bacterial invasion, it's a sign of your body effectively at work. But when these fires burn too long, they can contribute extensively to lifestyle diseases such as arthritis, heart diseases, and a plethora of autoimmune disorders.

This subtle systemic reaction might start as something as small and often dismissed as fatigue or a sore joint but could potentially escalate to affect your overall well-being. That's why understanding the underlying causes and knowing how to effectively manage it, is your first line of defense.

Throughout this chapter, we will delve into what sparks inflammation—from dietary triggers to environmental factors—and how these influences could be silently disrupting your health. With each page, you will gain insights into recognizing the signs your body might be showing you, signaling an inflammatory response. It's akin to learning a new language spoken solely by your own body. Once the dialogue begins, and you start to connect the dots between how you feel and what you are feeding your body, adjustments can be made. Real, tangible improvements beckon on the horizon of informed dietary choices.

Thus, understanding inflammation is not merely an academic pursuit; it's a practical, daily commitment to steering your life toward a healthier path. The knowledge you gain here aims to empower you to make such transformations with confidence and clarity.

1. What Is Inflammation? Causes and Triggers

Imagine your body as a highly sophisticated defense system. Just as a fire alarm detects smoke, your immune system detects health threats and reacts. This protective mechanism, known as inflammation, can, when under control, be your savior—swiftly dealing with injuries and infections. But what happens when the alarm bells sound without cessation, reacting to threats that aren't as clear-cut as, say, a bacterial invasion?

Inflammation can be broadly categorized into two types: acute and chronic. Acute inflammation is the type you are likely most familiar with—an immediate response to an injury or infection, often visible and certainly noticeable. It happens as a part of the body's natural healing process.

Conversely, chronic inflammation is the quieter, more insidious type that can lurk for years without overt symptoms.

Picture this as if your body's defense system were constantly on, even when you're not under attack. This maladaptation can lead to our immune system gradually turning on our own tissues, mistaking them for foreign invaders. Diseases such as arthritis, heart disease, and various autoimmune disorders often find their roots here, in the soils of chronic, unresolved inflammation.

Root Causes and Triggers of Chronic Inflammation

Understanding what triggers inflammation is crucial. It's similar to understanding what foods you're allergic to—you can avoid major discomfort by simply not consuming them.

Dietary Influences

For starters, our modern diet is a significant trigger. Foods high in sugar and saturated fats can provoke inflammatory responses. On the flip side, certain foods like fruits, vegetables, nuts, and fatty fish have natural anti-inflammatory properties. It's not just about what you eat, though; it's also how this food communicates with your body's metabolic and immune responses.

Environmental Factors

Environmental toxins also play a role. Consider how pollution or exposure to cigarette smoke can wreak havoc on your body. These toxins can trigger inflammation as your body attempts to fend off these perceived threats.

Chronic Stress

Chronic stress tells another tale of inflammation. Elevated stress levels affect your body in ways that might surprise you. Hormonal imbalances triggered by stress can prompt an inflammatory response. Picture your body in a continual state of fight or flight—a state in which it mistakenly views itself as perpetually under attack.

Gut Health

The health of your gut microbiome is another critical piece of the inflammation puzzle. An imbalance in this gut flora can lead to a weakened intestinal lining, allowing bacteria and toxins to enter the bloodstream, which may trigger inflammation. A balanced diet rich in fiber, healthy fats, and nutrients supports a robust microbiome, holding inflammatory responses at bay.

Physical Activity

Physical activity, or rather the lack of it, also contributes to chronic inflammation. Regular movement and exercise help manage weight, improve blood flow, and modulate various metabolic hormones that can naturally reduce inflammation.

From Ignorance to Awareness: Recognizing Inflammatory Responses

Recognizing the signs of inflammation is key to managing it. Often, they might manifest in ways that seem unrelated. It could be as subtle as feeling overly fatigued, experiencing inexplicable body aches, or something as persistent as having digestive issues.

Health is often spoken of as something one must monitor and control minutely, but such views can be daunting. Understanding inflammation and its triggers is less about vigilant control and more about gentle awareness. It involves tuning into your body's signals, understanding what they mean, and knowing how you can respond most effectively.

Strategic Steps Toward Managing and Reducing Inflammation

Managing and reducing inflammation begins with adjusting lifestyle habits, particularly diet. Incorporating anti-inflammatory foods is not just about choosing to eat certain foods over others; it's a shift toward a balanced, health-supportive pattern of eating.

Maintaining regular physical activity isn't just essential for weight management—it's an instrumental part of circulating anti-inflammatory compounds through your body and strengthening immune function.

Managing stress is also non-negotiable. Whether it's through mindfulness practices, yoga, or ensuring adequate sleep, reducing stress levels can significantly decrease inflammation.

Lastly, consider environmental factors. Minimizing exposure to pollutants and irritants is a responsible way to lower your inflammatory response. Whether it's choosing a smoke-free environment or opting for cleaner, less polluted areas to live and work, every little decision counts.

A Harmonized Approach

As you explore the maze of factors that influence inflammation, remember that the pathways to inflammation are as complex and interconnected as the solutions are supportive and multifaceted. Understanding what inflammation truly is and what triggers it in your life is not about fear-mongering—it's about empowering yourself with knowledge to make informed, health-promoting decisions every day.

The journey to managing inflammation doesn't demand perfection. It asks for awareness, patience, and small, perpetual steps towards what works uniquely for your body. As we unpack these themes further in the following sections, cultivating a balanced, inflammation-conscious lifestyle will increasingly appear not just feasible, but highly rewarding.

2. SYMPTOMS AND HEALTH RISKS

When inflammation becomes a regular visitor in your body, it rarely knocks loudly enough at first for us to notice right away. Its whispers through subtle symptoms might often be brushed off as the banalities of busy lives—tiredness at the end of a long day, stiff joints in the morning, or a persistent niggle in the gut.

Gradually, however, these whispers can become a cacophony that disrupts life in glaringly obvious ways. Understanding these symptoms and recognizing the potential health risks associated with prolonged inflammation is critical in turning down the volume and reasserting control over your health.

Recognizing the Symptoms

The first and often the most ignored symptoms of chronic inflammation are fatigue and pain. Unlike the acute pain that accompanies a cut or injury which is sharp and localized, the discomfort caused by chronic inflammation is often diffuse and lingering. It might manifest as backache, muscle aches, or joint pain. These are the kinds of aches that you can't quite pinpoint but are pervasive enough to affect your day-to-day activities.

Another frequent sign is persistent digestive issues. Whether it's bloating, diarrhea, constipation, or gastric discomfort, these gut-related symptoms are your body signaling trouble. The gastrointestinal tract is closely tied to your immune system, and when inflammatory responses are misfired, the gut is often one of the first sites of impact.

Skin changes are another indicator of chronic inflammation. Conditions like eczema, psoriasis, and persistent acne are visible markers that the body's inflammatory response may be in overdrive. Your skin, the largest organ in your body, acts like a billboard displaying messages from the inside.

Furthermore, frequent infections, weight fluctuations, and ongoing feelings of fatigue or malaise are indicative of a compromised immune system affected by inflammation. When your immune system is engaged non-stop, it becomes less capable of managing invaders effectively, leading to both minor and more severe health implications.

Health Risks Linked to Chronic Inflammation

The risks associated with long-term inflammation stretch across nearly every major organ system in the body. It's a root cause linked to numerous diseases, many of which are among the leading causes of disability and death worldwide.

Heart Disease

Chronic inflammation is closely linked with several pathologies of the cardiovascular system, including heart attacks and strokes. It contributes to the buildup of arterial plaque, and these plaques' potential rupture could lead to severe outcomes. The inner walls of the arteries swell due to inflammatory responses, which reduce the overall width through which blood can flow, escalating the potential for blockages.

Type 2 Diabetes

Inflammation also plays a significant role in insulin resistance, which can lead to Type 2 Diabetes. When your body's cells become less responsive to insulin due to inflammatory signals, your pancreas struggles to keep up with the increased demand for insulin, eventually leading to sugar imbalances in your bloodstream.

Autoimmune Diseases

In cases like rheumatoid arthritis, systemic lupus erythematosus, and others, the body's immune system, driven by chronic inflammation, begins attacking its tissues, mistaking them for external threats. This self-destructive process can lead to widespread inflammation and varying degrees of organ and tissue damage.

Neurological Decline

Emerging evidence links inflammation with an increased risk of neurodegenerative diseases like Alzheimer's disease and other dementias. Chronic inflammation might contribute to neuronal damage and death, exacerbating these conditions' development and progression.

Connecting the Dots Between Symptoms and Risks

The journey from ignoring a persistently irritable gut to dealing with a serious health diagnosis can be slow and insidious, making it crucial to connect these dots early. Monitoring the signs and understanding their potential ramifications enables you to advocate for early interventions, potentially averting the risk of severe diseases.

Ultimately, recognizing these symptoms and understanding the associated risks isn't meant to alarm you—it's meant to empower you. Knowledge here acts as a tool, giving you the leverage to make changes where they're most needed, whether that's adjusting your diet, enhancing your exercise routine, managing stress, or seeking medical advice.

Given that every individual's body communicates in its nuances, the symptoms and their intensities can vary. However, the fundamental response by the body through inflammatory pathways is a shared commonality. By reading your body's signals through a lens informed by knowledge, the management of inflammation can transition from reactive to proactive, paving the way for not just a healthier lifestyle but potentially a longer, more fulfilling life.

Chapter 2: Food List

Imagine you're in the grocery store, standing in the produce aisle. Your cart is empty, your list is in hand, but where do you start? This chapter isn't just a list; it's your personal tour guide through the world of anti-inflammatory eating, where every choice you make can bring you a step closer to a healthier, livelier you.

In the vast ocean of food options, it becomes essential to distinguish between those that can fuel inflammation, akin to throwing gasoline on a fire, and those that can help extinguish it. The distinction is critical because what we consume directly influences our body's inflammatory processes. It's not just about avoiding bad foods, but about embracing those powerful, nutrient-rich foods that can not only reduce inflammation but also enhance our overall health.

Think of anti-inflammatory foods as your body's best friends—they whisper calm into the chaotic conversations happening at the cellular level. These foods are rich in antioxidants, vitamins, and minerals which soothe your systems rather than provoking them. Here, the focus is twofold: identifying these treasures and understanding how they contribute to easing your body's inflammatory response.

We'll explore the vibrant colors and textures of fruits and vegetables like berries, broccoli, and leafy greens that aren't just pleasing to the eye but are packed with phytochemicals and antioxidants. We'll delve into the world of whole grains, where fiber does more than just aid digestion; it fosters a gut environment that dampens inflammatory signals. Then, there's the power of omega-3 fatty acids found abundantly in fatty fish and flaxseeds, known for their remarkable ability to quell inflammation.

This journey through anti-inflammatory foods isn't about restricting your diet—it's about enriching it. It's about making choices that delight your palate while simultaneously caring for your body. As we traverse this landscape of foods, remember that each has a role, a potential to contribute positively to your health. While these foods are your allies in fighting inflammation, their incorporation into your daily diet should feel less like a mandate and more like a series of enjoyable, health-affirming selections.

1. Foods That Fuel Inflammation

Let's begin our exploration into the often overlooked, yet immensely impactful world of foods that fuel inflammation. These are not just foods; they are the silent aggravators lurking in your kitchen, masquerading as comfort, often leading to distress in your body's systems.

Often, the story of inflammatory foods is a tale of modern dietary patterns, where processing, preserving, and preparing take precedence over natural nutrition. The fundamental elements include refined sugars, trans fats, and excessive omega-6 fatty acids, found abundantly in many staples of the Western diet. As we peel back the layers, it becomes evident how these items, convenient and pleasing to the palate as they may be, contribute to ongoing inflammation—a root cause of various chronic health issues.

Imagine a typical day: starting with a breakfast of pastries or sugary cereals, a lunch featuring a burger with a side of fries, and dinner composed of a large serving of pasta with a few token vegetables. While tasty, these meals often have a high glycemic index, rich in refined carbs and sugars that spike your blood sugar levels and, in turn, your body's inflammatory response.

Refined sugar—found in sodas, most processed foods, and desserts—is akin to throwing fuel on the flames of inflammation. When you consume these sugars, your body releases cytokines, inflammatory messengers that contribute to the overall inflammatory burden.

But it's not just sugar. Let's talk about trans fats. These are found in some margarines, fast foods, and various baked goods. Trans fats are notorious not just for their role in heart disease but also as catalysts for inflammation. They are like unwelcome guests who stubbornly refuse to leave, disrupting your body's natural metabolic harmony and igniting inflammatory responses.

Shifting focus, consider omega-6 fatty acids. While essential, an imbalance favoring omega-6s over omega-3s in your diet can lead to inflammation. Commonly used vegetable oils like soybean, corn, and sunflower are high in omega-6 fatty acids. In moderation and within a balanced diet, they're generally fine, but the typical dietary patterns tip the scales towards an excess, fostering an environment ripe for inflammatory reactions.

Another aspect of our modern diet contributing to this inflammatory milieu includes certain additives—preservatives, flavor enhancers, and artificial colors. These components are often ignored because they appear in such minute quantities. However, their constant presence in our diet can add up, contributing subtly yet significantly to long-term health issues.

But what about gluten and dairy? For many, these are staples, but for others, they are triggers. Gluten, a protein found in wheat, barley, and rye, can cause inflammation in susceptible individuals, especially those with celiac disease or gluten sensitivity. Dairy, meanwhile, can also be inflammatory for those with a lactose intolerance or a sensitivity to casein, a protein found in milk. Here, it's the immune system's response to these proteins that sparks an inflammatory process, which if continually triggered, can lead to more systemic issues.

The key takeaway is not to shun these foods entirely—at least not without cause. It's about recognizing the trigger points for your body. What fuels inflammation in one might be perfectly fine for another. The journey to understanding the role of these foods in your health begins with awareness followed by moderated, mindful consumption.

Reducing these inflammatory foods doesn't imply a life of bland meals or significant dietary sacrifices. On the contrary, it opens a new chapter where wholesome, anti-inflammatory foods enrich your diet, bringing balance and vibrancy. This switch, though initially challenging, can be immensely rewarding, leading not just to reduced inflammation, but also to a revitalized, energetic life.

The narrative of inflammatory foods is not simply about avoidance; it's about transformation and empowerment through your diet. Understanding the impact of your food choices sets the stage for this positive change. By recognizing and reducing the presence of these inflammatory foods, you pave the way for a healthier, more enjoyable eating experience that supports your body's natural defenses against inflammation, bolstering your overall well-being.

2. ANTI-INFLAMMATORY FOODS

As we transition from understanding the foods that fuel inflammation, let's illuminate the brighter side of the spectrum—the vibrant, nourishing world of anti-inflammatory foods. These are not just ingredients but powerful allies in your journey towards a healthier, more vibrant life.

Picture a lush green forest, brimming with life. Each plant, each leaf, and fruit has a role, contributing to the health and balance of the ecosystem. Similarly, anti-inflammatory foods work synergistically to create a balanced, health-sustaining diet that nurtures your body, reducing inflammation and enhancing overall well-being.

Begin with the colorful guardians of health: fruits and vegetables. Berries, for instance, are jewels of the culinary world, brimming with antioxidants such as vitamin C and flavonoids. Blueberries, strawberries, and raspberries aren't just delightful to the taste but are powerhouses of nutrients, fighting against the oxidative stress that can trigger inflammation.

Then there are the mighty greens—spinach, kale, and broccoli—each leaf packed with vitamins A, C, and K, along with minerals like magnesium. These aren't just nutrients; they are the warriors against inflammation, ensuring your body's balance is maintained.

Moreover, consider the humble beetroot, with its deep crimson hue, a telltale sign of betalains, which possess potent antioxidant properties. Similarly, the often-overlooked spice, turmeric, contains curcumin, a compound well-studied for its anti-inflammatory effects. When combined with black pepper, whose piperine enhances curcumin absorption, its efficacy in combatting inflammation is significantly boosted.

Now, let's touch upon the fatty fish like salmon, mackerel, and sardines, rich in omega-3 fatty acids. Unlike the omega-6 fatty acids predominant in the modern diet, omega-3s help reduce the levels of inflammatory eicosanoids and cytokines. Regular consumption of these fish can lead to a decreased risk of chronic diseases such as heart disease, arthritis, and more, showcasing the critical role diet plays in managing inflammation.

Nuts and seeds also have a part to play. Almonds, chia seeds, and flaxseeds are not only tasty snacks but also rich in ALA (alpha-linolenic acid), another type of omega-3 fatty acid. Including these in your diet means engaging in a daily ritual of reducing inflammation with every crunch.

Let's not overlook the essentials—olive oil, a staple of the Mediterranean diet, renowned for its high levels of oleocanthal, which has properties similar to non-steroidal anti-inflammatory drugs. Integrating olive oil into your diet can be as simple as drizzling it over salad or using it as a base for sauces, making it a delicious way to enjoy its health benefits.

In the realm of flavors, spices like ginger and garlic also play significant roles. Ginger contains gingerol, which suppresses cytokines and chemokines before they can affect body tissues. Garlic, powered by diallyl disulfide, an anti-inflammatory compound, helps fight inflammation and potentially reduce the risk of arteriosclerosis.

Every sip matters too. Green tea, for instance, is admired globally not only for its calming qualities but also for its catechins—antioxidants that reduce inflammatory responses in the body. Similarly, theobromine in dark chocolate, when consumed in moderation, can support heart health by easing arterial inflammation.

Adopting a diet rich in these anti-inflammatory foods doesn't entail a complete overhaul of your eating habits overnight. Small, manageable integrations, like opting for a handful of nuts as a snack or choosing whole grains over refined ones, can significantly influence your body's inflammatory processes.

As we wrap up this vivid tour of anti-inflammatory foods, remember, it's not about rigid dietary restrictions but about making mindful, flavorful additions to your meals. Each fruit, each vegetable, each seed you choose comes with a promise—not just of good taste, but of health, vitality, and a vibrant life. These foods are not just ingredients; they are a testament to nature's power to heal, to restore, and to sustain. Through them, you wield the power to not only combat inflammation but to thrive.

CHAPTER 3: ESSENTIAL NUTRIENTS FOR REDUCING INFLAMMATION

Stepping into the world of anti-inflammatory nutrients feels a bit like unlocking a secret garden—each vitamin, mineral, and compound holds potential not just to soothe but to rejuvenate your body. Imagine these nutrients as your personal health allies, each one ready to support your journey towards a more vibrant, pain-free life. It's about transforming the way your body handles inflammation, turning the tide in your favor with every meal you enjoy.

Now, envision your body as a complex network of systems needing harmony and balance. Inflammation, when chronic, disrupts this balance, contributing to a range of health issues from fatigue to chronic pain. However, by infusing our diet with key nutrients, we can help restore this balance delicately and effectively. This chapter isn't just about listing these beneficial nutrients; it's about understanding how they weave their magic.

Let's take Omega-3 fatty acids, for example, renowned not only for their anti-inflammatory properties but also for their role in heart health and cognitive function. Found abundantly in fish like salmon and in plant sources such as flaxseeds, incorporating Omega-3s into your diet isn't just an act of healing, it's an investment in your overall well-being.

Similarly, antioxidants and phytochemicals guard your cells like vigilant sentinels, protecting them from the oxidative stress that fuels inflammation. Picture the vibrant colors of berries, the deep greens of spinach—these aren't just pleasing to the eye but are indicative of their rich antioxidant content.

And let's not forget about vitamins and minerals—each one playing a pivotal role. Vitamin D, often garnered from sunlight and fortified foods, helps modulate immune responses, a key aspect for managing inflammation. Magnesium, a natural relaxant, aids in muscle and nerve function and helps maintain normal immune function.

By the end of this chapter, you'll not only be familiar with these essential nutrients but will also have the know-how to incorporate them creatively and deliciously into your daily meals. This isn't just about eating away pain, it's about nourishing your body in a way that empowers it to heal and thrive. As we explore these nutrients in depth, remember, each step you take on this dietary journey brings you closer to a more balanced, health-optimized life.

1. VITAMINS AND MINERALS

In our quest to conquer inflammation through diet, vitamins and minerals play starring roles—a veritable cast of characters each contributing their unique strengths to restore and maintain our health. These elements are the unsung heroes, often overshadowed by more glamorous nutrients, yet without them, our bodies could not perform the complex biochemical processes required to reduce inflammation and promote healing.

Let's begin with Vitamin D, often hailed as the "sunshine vitamin." Besides its critical role in bone health, Vitamin D has impressive anti-inflammatory credentials. It modulates the immune system, which is pivotal because an overactive immune response is often the underlying cause of systemic inflammation. Consider the northern latitudes where sunshine is scarce; populations there often suffer from higher rates of certain autoimmune diseases. This is no coincidence—Vitamin D deficiency is linked to increased inflammation and an upsurge in immune-related disorders. Including Vitamin D rich foods like fatty fish, fortified dairy, or plant milk, and making sure to get some sun exposure can significantly alter your body's inflammatory response.

Then, there's the powerful antioxidant duo of Vitamin C and Vitamin E. Vitamin C does more than fend off the common cold—it also combats free radicals, the unstable molecules that exacerbate inflammation in the body. This water-soluble vitamin is abundant in citrus fruits, bell peppers, and dark leafy greens. It works synergistically with Vitamin E, a fat-soluble antioxidant, which protects cell membranes from oxidative stress. Vitamin E can be found in nuts, seeds, and whole grains—it's this protective quality that shields our cells from the inflammatory damage caused by free radicals.

Equally important for their anti-inflammatory effects are the B vitamins, particularly B6, B9 (folate), and B12. These vitamins play crucial roles in methylation—the process by which our bodies regulate gene expression and maintain the immune system. Low levels of these vitamins are associated with an increased inflammatory response. To ensure adequate intake, include a variety of animal products like fish and poultry, legumes, and leafy greens in your diet.

Magnesium deserves a special mention here. This mineral supports hundreds of biochemical reactions in the body, including those that control the immune response. Magnesium deficiency is notoriously common and can exacerbate inflammatory conditions. It calms the nervous system and reduces stress, which in turn can minimize the release of stress hormones that trigger inflammation. Foods rich in magnesium include almonds, spinach, and black beans, and integrating these into your meals can be a straightforward way to boost your intake.

Another mineral, zinc, influences inflammation through its critical role in immune function and cell growth. It helps the immune system fight off invading bacteria and viruses, a direct benefit in controlling sources of inflammation that can go unnoticed at first. The body also needs zinc to produce protein and DNA, the genetic material in all cells. While it's commonly taken in supplement form to fend off colds, its natural forms are plentiful in meat, shellfish, and legumes.

Selenium, though often less talked about, connects antioxidant activity with immune function. This trace mineral enhances the efficacy of antioxidants, helping to prevent the cellular damage associated with chronic inflammation. It's a potent ally found naturally in Brazil nuts, seafood, and mushrooms.

While discussing vitamins and minerals, it's also worth considering how they work not just in isolation but synergistically. A diet rich in a broad spectrum of vitamins and minerals—obtained from a variety of sources—ensures a stronger, more resilient anti-inflammatory response. Vitamins and minerals interact intricately: Vitamin E is better absorbed with Vitamin C, magnesium needs vitamin D to be effectively utilized by the body, and zinc performs optimally in the presence of adequate fatty acid levels. It's less about focusing on one nutrient at a time and more about maintaining a balance that supports overall health.

We've seen that an anti-inflammatory diet isn't a restricted diet—it's diversified, rich in colorful fruits and vegetables, lean proteins, whole grains, nuts, and seeds. Each meal provides more than mere sustenance: it's a cocktail of chemicals crucial for health, designed by nature to work together, reducing inflammation and promoting healing.

By choosing your foods wisely and ensuring you're not inadvertently consuming items that could deplete these crucial nutrients, you set the stage for a body well-equipped to fight inflammation. For instance, excessive alcohol consumption can decrease the absorption of several B vitamins; similarly, a diet high in processed foods can significantly reduce magnesium levels.

Remember, the journey to an anti-inflammatory lifestyle doesn't need to be a solo voyage. Consulting with healthcare providers to measure your levels of these essential nutrients can be an enlightening part of your journey. They can provide further guidance on how to balance dietary intake and supplements in a way that meets your personal health needs, ensuring that you're not just following a diet but embracing a healthier life through informed, nutrition-conscious decisions.

In essence, understanding and incorporating a broad spectrum of vitamins and minerals into our daily diet is key to managing and mitigating inflammation naturally. As we move through this book, think of each nutritional choice as a step towards a healthier, more vibrant you.

2. OMEGA-3 FATTY ACIDS

Imagine the body as a complex ecosystem that thrives on balance and harmony. Among the myriad nutrients essential for maintaining this balance, Omega-3 fatty acids stand out as powerful agents of anti-inflammatory action, playing crucial roles in not just combating inflammation but also enhancing overall health. These fatty acids are akin to high-grade oil that keeps the machinery of our bodies running smoothly, ensuring that inflammatory responses don't become chronic or detrimental.

Omega-3s are a group of essential fatty acids that the body cannot produce on its own, thus they must be obtained through diet. The three main types are ALA (alpha-linolenic acid), found in plant oils, and EPA (eicosapentaenoic acid) and DHA (docosahexaenoic acid), primarily found in marine sources. The journey of these fatty acids through the body illustrates their vital role in reducing inflammation and supporting health in several significant ways.

Firstly, EPA and DHA are well-known for their contribution to heart health, improving cardiovascular functions, and reducing the likelihood of heart diseases. But their benefits extend much further—they modulate the inflammatory processes by interfering with the production of inflammatory eicosanoids and cytokines. In simpler terms, they help to turn off the fires of chronic inflammation that can smolder within the body, potentially leading to various diseases.

The relationship between omega-3 fatty acids and inflammation is a dynamic one. They are incorporated into cell membranes and are involved in the cell signaling processes that govern the body's inflammatory response. By altering cell membrane composition, omega-3s enhance the body's ability to mediate inflammation and aid in the repair and recovery of tissues.

EPA and DHA also play a protective role in brain health, influencing the brain's structure and signaling systems. They are essential for maintaining the fluidity of cell membranes, necessary for proper cell function and communication. This includes supporting cognitive functions and potentially reducing the risk of mental decline as we age.

For mental health, researchers have found a correlation between higher levels of omega-3 intake and a decrease in depressive symptoms. This is thought to be because of omega-3's ability to enhance brain function and reduce inflammation, which is often elevated in mood disorders.

Additionally, these fatty acids are pivotal in supporting the immune system. By regulating the body's immune response, they ensure that it does not overreact, which can lead to autoimmune diseases, where the body mistakenly attacks its own tissues.

Considering all these benefits, incorporating omega-3 fatty acids into one's diet is a central component of any strategy aimed at fighting inflammation. Rich marine sources like salmon, mackerel, and sardines are excellent sources of EPA and DHA. For vegetarians or those who prefer plant-based sources, flaxseeds, chia seeds, and walnuts are good sources of ALA, which the body can convert to EPA and DHA, though the conversion rate is low. This underscores the need for diverse dietary sources or, in some cases, supplements to meet the recommended intake.

Navigating the world of supplements, particularly omega-3s, requests careful consideration. While they can be a practical solution for those who find it challenging to receive enough from their diet, it's crucial to choose high-quality products to avoid contaminants such as heavy metals often associated with fish oils. Consulting with a healthcare provider can help determine the need and the right dosage.

One should not underestimate the potential of dietary changes. Consistently choosing foods rich in omega-3s can contribute substantially to reducing inflammation naturally without the side effects that often accompany pharmacological interventions.

In essence, understanding omega-3 fatty acids unravels a fundamental truth about our health - enduring health is not merely the absence of disease but the presence of vital nutrients that continually enable, enhance, and sustain our body's natural defense systems. As we integrate more omega-3-rich foods into our diet, we provide our bodies with the essential tools needed not just to fight inflammation but to thrive. This dynamic, intriguing interplay between what we consume and how our bodies operate is not merely a footnote in our personal health narrative—it is, perhaps, its very foundation.

3. ANTIOXIDANTS AND PHYTOCHEMICALS

Diving into the vibrant world of antioxidants and phytochemicals is akin to exploring a vivid palette of nature's best defenses against inflammation. These compounds, abundant in fruits, vegetables, grains, and nuts, are not only the source of the brilliant colors and varied flavors in foods but are also crucial in combatting inflammation and enhancing overall health. They represent a powerful arsenal equipped by nature to fight against oxidative stress, a common precursor to inflammation.

Antioxidants, as the name suggests, counteract oxidation—a chemical reaction that can produce free radicals, leading to cell damage. It's this damage, if unchecked, that can lead to chronic inflammation and subsequently a host of other diseases including arthritis, heart disease, and even cancer. Think of antioxidants as the body's own firefighting team, quelling the flames of inflammation at a molecular level before they can cause harm.

Phytochemicals, a broad category encompassing thousands of beneficial chemicals in plants, also play a significant role in managing inflammation. While not traditionally categorized as nutrients essential for survival, they help to improve human health and resilience in many ways. They orchestrate a complex dance of cellular signaling, immune function, and antioxidant defense to maintain the health of tissues and organs.

One of the most lauded groups of phytochemicals are the flavonoids, found in fruits, vegetables, chocolates, and even beverages like tea and wine. Flavonoids are potent anti-inflammatory agents, capable of inhibiting enzymes that produce inflammatory molecules and modulating signaling pathways that reduce risk and severity of diseases. For example, the flavonoid quercetin, abundant in onions and apples, has been found to significantly dampen inflammation in numerous studies. Carotenoids, another family of phytochemicals, give yellow, orange, and red fruits and vegetables their vibrant colors. Beta-carotene, lycopene, and lutein are types of carotenoids that have strong antioxidant properties. Beta-carotene, converted into vitamin A in the body, supports immune function and plays a protective role in eye health and skin. Lycopene, prevalent in tomatoes, has been linked to a reduced risk of certain types of cancer, particularly prostate cancer.

Sulforaphane, a sulfur-rich compound found in cruciferous vegetables like broccoli and Brussels sprouts, activates a variety of antioxidant and detoxification enzymes that protect against molecular damage. Numerous studies suggest that it also has potent anti-inflammatory properties, influencing gene expression to favor anti-inflammatory states over pro-inflammatory ones.

Further venturing into the realm of these cellular protectors unveils another group of phytochemicals known as polyphenols. Found in green tea, grapes, olive oil, and whole grains, polyphenols have been associated with a reduced risk of several chronic diseases due to their ability to mitigate oxidative stress and soothe inflammation. The benefits of green tea, largely attributed to its polyphenols, include the inhibition of inflammatory pathways and mechanisms that can lead to cancer development and progression.

Integrating a diet rich in these antioxidants and phytochemicals doesn't just mitigate inflammation. It fortifies the body's defenses, enriching cell health, safeguarding against environmental pollutants, and slowing down aging processes. Rich, varied, and natural sources of antioxidants and phytochemicals can transform meals into therapeutic remedies healing the body from within.

But the protective impact of antioxidants and phytochemicals is not merely contingent upon consumption. Factors like food preparation techniques can influence the levels of these beneficial compounds. For example, gently cooking tomatoes enhances the bioavailability of lycopene, while overly boiling vegetables can lead to significant loss of beneficial antioxidants. Thus, optimally harnessing the benefits of these compounds involves thoughtful dietary choices and preparation methods.

This complex interplay between antioxidants, phytochemicals, and inflammation implies more than just eating a few fruits and vegetables sporadically. It calls for a conscious, consistent approach to diet, tailored to imbue your body with these invaluable compounds regularly. Including a spectrum of colorful plants in every meal not only paints your plate with enticing hues but also layers your immune system with necessary tools to combat inflammation and thereby reduce risks of disease.

Understanding and utilizing the myriad benefits of antioxidants and phytochemicals thus constructs more than a barrier against disease—it designs a comprehensive blueprint for robust health.

CHAPTER 6: BREAKFAST RECIPES

Starting each day with the right meal not only sets the tone for your morning but also for your overall well-being. That's why breakfast is often lauded as the most important meal of the day, especially when we're focusing on reducing inflammation and boosting our health. Our journey toward a more serene and vibrant lifestyle begins the moment we wake up; hence, incorporating anti-inflammatory foods into our breakfast can transform our day from the very first bite.

Imagine waking up to a meal that energizes without increasing inflammation, using ingredients that are both nurturing and delightful. The recipes in this chapter are designed to introduce you to a variety of flavors and nutrients that ward off inflammation, with each dish crafted to integrate seamlessly into your busy morning routine. Whether you have just a few minutes to spare or can indulge in a leisurely morning meal, you'll find options to suit your schedule and palate.

For those mornings when time is not on our side, I've included quick smoothies packed with omega-3s and colorful bowls of mixed fruits topped with anti-inflammatory seeds. For a more leisurely breakfast, you can delve into dishes like turmeric-infused scrambled eggs, which not only provide a vibrant color and flavor but also significant anti-inflammatory benefits. Each recipe aims to please the taste buds while offering the nutritional backbone your body needs to combat inflammation.

What makes these breakfast choices so vital? They consist of ingredients like blueberries rich in antioxidants, spinach overflowing with magnesium, and nuts loaded with healthy fats known to help reduce biochemical markers of inflammation. This is not just food; this is your first step each day towards a healthier life.

Through these recipes, my goal is to introduce you to the potent combination of enjoyment and wellness. A delightful breakfast that fits into your hectic schedule is completely achievable and can be tremendously beneficial. Let these meals lift your spirit and health as you start your day, empowering you to face whatever comes with renewed energy and a calm body.

GOLDEN TURMERIC MORNING ELIXIR

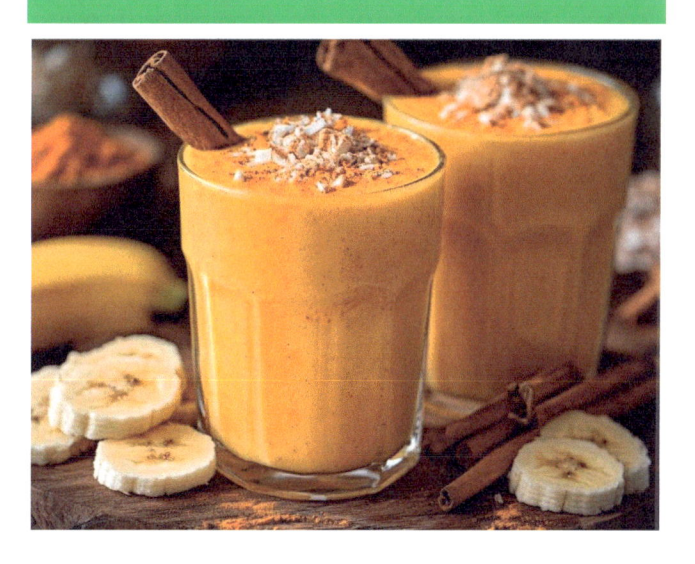

Preparation Time: 5 min.
Cooking Time: none

Mode of Cooking: Blending

Servings: 2 Serv.

Ingredients:

- 1 cup coconut water
- ½ banana
- 1 Tbsp ground turmeric
- 1 Tbsp ground flaxseed
- 1 tsp cinnamon
- 1 tsp fresh ginger, grated
- 1 Tbsp honey
- Ice cubes

Directions:

1. Place all ingredients in the blender
2. Blend until smooth
3. Pour into glasses and serve immediately

Tips:

- Add a pinch of black pepper to increase turmeric absorption
- Use frozen banana for a creamier texture

Nutritional Values: Calories: 120, Fat: 2g, Carbs: 25g, Protein: 2g, Sugar: 15g, Sodium: 40 mg, Potassium: 200 mg, Cholesterol: 0 mg

GREEN DETOX POWER SMOOTHIE

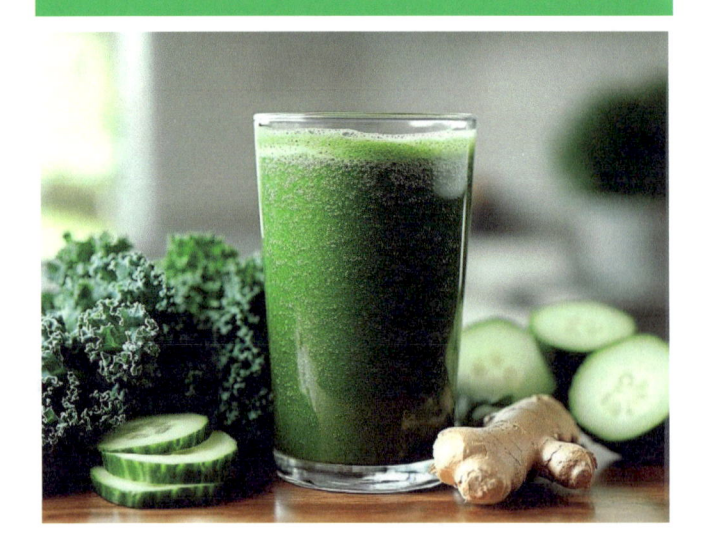

Preparation Time: 7 min.

Cooking Time: none

Mode of Cooking: Blending

Servings: 2

Ingredients:

- 1 cup kale leaves, stems removed
- ½ green apple, cored and chopped
- ½ cucumber, sliced
- ¼ cup parsley leaves
- 2 Tbsp lemon juice
- 1 Tbsp ginger, peeled and grated
- 1 cup coconut water
- 1 tsp spirulina powder
- Ice cubes

Directions:

1. Add kale, apple, cucumber, parsley, lemon juice, ginger, coconut water, and spirulina powder to a blender
2. Blend until smooth
3. Pour over ice and serve chilled

Tips:

- Incorporate a scoop of plant-based protein powder for a protein boost
- Peel and freeze apple slices beforehand for extra chill and thickness in the smoothie

Nutritional Values: Calories: 90, Fat: 1g, Carbs: 20g, Protein: 3g, Sugar: 8g, Sodium: 50 mg, Potassium: 300 mg, Cholesterol: 0 mg

BLUEBERRY AVOCADO BLISS SMOOTHIE

Preparation Time: 5 min.

Cooking Time: none

Mode of Cooking: Blending

Servings: 2

Ingredients:
- 1 ripe avocado, pitted and scooped
- 1 cup fresh blueberries
- 1 cup spinach leaves
- 1 Tbsp chia seeds
- 1 Tbsp lemon juice
- 1 cup almond milk
- 1 tsp honey
- Ice cubes

Directions:
1. Combine avocado, blueberries, spinach, chia seeds, lemon juice, almond milk, and honey in a blender
2. Blend until creamy and smooth
3. Add ice and blend briefly until chilled

Tips:
- Use organic blueberries to minimize pesticide intake
- Substitute honey with agave for a vegan option
- Spinach can be replaced with kale for variety

Nutritional Values: Calories: 220, Fat: 12g, Carbs: 28g, Protein: 4g, Sugar: 12g, Sodium: 30 mg, Potassium: 500 mg, Cholesterol: 0 mg

SPICED BERRY METABOLISM BOOSTER

Preparation Time: 6 min.
Cooking Time: none
Mode of Cooking: Blending
Servings: 2

Ingredients:
- 1 cup frozen mixed berries
- 1 cup unsweetened Greek yogurt
- 1 Tbsp ground flaxseed
- ½ tsp cinnamon
- ¼ tsp nutmeg
- 1 Tbsp almond butter
- 1 tsp honey
- 1 cup almond milk

Directions:
1. Blend all ingredients together until smooth
2. Serve immediately in chilled glasses

Tips:
- Experiment with different types of berries for flavor variation
- Add a scoop of vanilla protein powder for a protein enhancement
- Cinnamon can be increased according to taste preference

Nutritional Values: Calories: 160, Fat: 9g, Carbs: 18g, Protein: 8g, Sugar: 10g, Sodium: 60 mg, Potassium: 250 mg, Cholesterol: 5 mg

PINEAPPLE GINGER IMMUNE BOOSTER

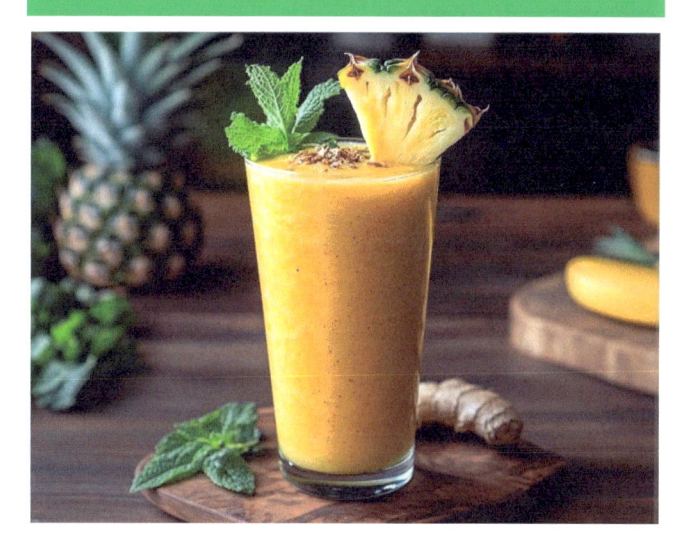

Preparation Time: 5 min.
Cooking Time: none

Mode of Cooking: Blending

Servings: 2

Ingredients:

- 1 cup pineapple chunks
- ½ banana
- 1 Tbsp freshly grated ginger
- 1 cup kale leaves
- 1 Tbsp lemon juice
- 1 tsp turmeric powder
- 1 cup water
- Ice cubes

Directions:

1. Blend pineapple, banana, ginger, kale, lemon juice, turmeric, and water until smooth
2. Add ice and blend until frosty
3. Serve immediately

Tips:

- Use fresh pineapple for the best flavor and nutrient content
- Optional: add a teaspoon of honey for extra sweetness if desired
- Ginger quantity can be adjusted for spice level preference

Nutritional Values: Calories: 130, Fat: 1g, Carbs: 31g, Protein: 2g, Sugar: 20g, Sodium: 20 mg, Potassium: 400 mg, Cholesterol: 0 mg

TURMERIC GINGER CHIA PUDDING

Preparation Time: 15 min

Cooking Time: none

Mode of Cooking: No Cooking

Servings: 2

Ingredients:

- 1 C. coconut milk
- 3 Tbsp chia seeds
- 1 tsp ground turmeric
- ½ tsp ground ginger
- 1 Tbsp honey
- ½ tsp vanilla extract
- Pinch of black pepper

Directions:

1. Combine coconut milk, chia seeds, turmeric, ginger, honey, vanilla extract, and black pepper in a bowl
2. Stir thoroughly until well mixed
3. Cover and refrigerate overnight to allow chia seeds to swell and absorb liquids

Tips:

- Serve with a sprinkle of grated coconut for an extra tropical twist
- Black pepper enhances the absorption of turmeric, boosting its anti-inflammatory properties
- Opt for raw, organic honey for additional antioxidants

Nutritional Values: Calories: 295, Fat: 19g, Carbs: 25g, Protein: 5g, Sugar: 12g, Sodium: 15 mg, Potassium: 406 mg, Cholesterol: 0 mg

OMEGA BOOSTER SMOOTHIE BOWL

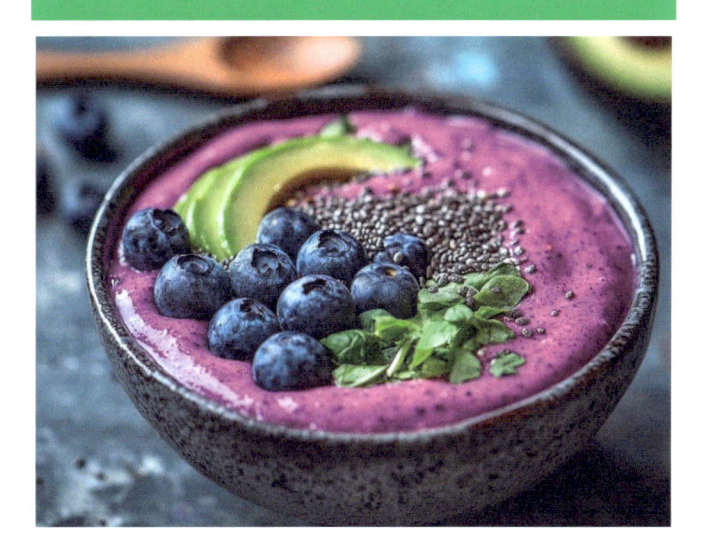

Preparation Time: 10 min
Cooking Time: none
Mode of Cooking: Blending
Servings: 1
Ingredients:
- 1 C. spinach
- ½ avocado
- ½ C. frozen blueberries
- 1 Tbsp flaxseeds
- 1 C. almond milk
- 1 Tbsp chia seeds
- 1 tsp honey

Directions:
1. Place spinach, avocado, blueberries, flaxseeds, almond milk, chia seeds, and honey in a blender
2. Blend on high until smooth
3. Pour into a bowl and garnish with your favorite seeds and nuts

Tips:
- Adding a scoop of protein powder increases satiety and muscle repair
- Use frozen fruit to make the smoothie bowl more refreshing and thick
- Spinach and flaxseeds are excellent sources of Omega-3 which helps reduce inflammation

Nutritional Values: Calories: 340, Fat: 19g, Carbs: 40g, Protein: 8g, Sugar: 15g, Sodium: 110 mg, Potassium: 578 mg, Cholesterol: 0 mg

SAVORY QUINOA BREAKFAST BOWL

Preparation Time: 20 min
Cooking Time: 25 min
Mode of Cooking: Boiling and Sautéing
Servings: 2
Ingredients:
- 1 C. quinoa
- 2 C. water
- 1 Tbsp olive oil
- 1 clove garlic, minced
- 1 small onion, diced
- ½ red bell pepper, diced
- 1 C. kale, chopped
- 2 eggs
- Salt and pepper to taste

Directions:
1. Rinse quinoa under cold water
2. In a saucepan, bring quinoa and water to a boil, cover, reduce heat, and simmer for 15 min until water is absorbed
3. Heat olive oil in a skillet, sauté garlic, onion, and bell pepper until soft
4. Add kale and cooked quinoa, sauté for another 5 min
5. In another pan, fry eggs to your liking

6. Serve quinoa veggie mix topped with fried egg

Tips:

- Experiment with different vegetables like spinach or zucchini for variety
- Quinoa is full of protein and fiber, aiding digestion and reducing inflammation
- Adding a dash of turmeric to the veggies while cooking can enhance the anti-inflammatory benefits

Nutritional Values: Calories: 410, Fat: 15g, Carbs: 55g, Protein: 18g, Sugar: 4g, Sodium: 70 mg, Potassium: 712 mg, Cholesterol: 186 mg

Berry Antioxidant Oatmeal

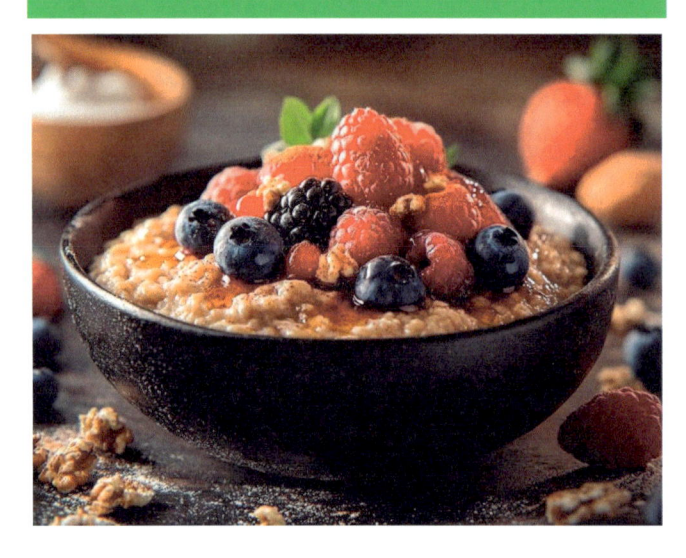

Preparation Time: 10 min
Cooking Time: 15 min
Mode of Cooking: Boiling
Servings: 2
Ingredients:

- 1 C. rolled oats
- 2 C. water
- ½ tsp cinnamon
- 1 C. mixed berries (strawberries, blueberries, raspberries)
- 1 Tbsp chopped walnuts
- 1 Tbsp honey

Directions:

1. In a medium saucepan, bring water to a boil
2. Add oats and cinnamon, reduce heat to low and simmer for 10 to 15 min, stirring occasionally
3. Once cooked, stir in the berries and honey
4. Serve topped with walnuts

Tips:

- Include a dollop of Greek yogurt for added protein and creaminess
- Berries are high in antioxidants, which combat free radicals and reduce inflammation
- Sprinkle ground flaxseeds on top for an Omega-3 boost

Nutritional Values: Calories: 270, Fat: 9g, Carbs: 44g, Protein: 6g, Sugar: 12g, Sodium: 10 mg, Potassium: 222 mg, Cholesterol: 0 mg

Sweet Potato & Kale Hash

Preparation Time: 10 min
Cooking Time: 20 min
Mode of Cooking: Sautéing
Servings: 2
Ingredients:

- 1 large sweet potato, diced
- 1 Tbsp olive oil
- 1 C. kale, chopped
- 1 small onion, diced
- 2 cloves garlic, minced
- Salt and pepper to taste

- ¼ tsp smoked paprika

Directions:

1. Heat olive oil in a large skillet over medium heat
2. Add diced sweet potato, season with salt, pepper, and smoked paprika, cook until they start to soften, about 10 min
3. Add onion and garlic, continue to cook for another 5 min
4. Add kale and cook until wilted and potatoes are fully tender

Tips:

- Serve with a poached egg on top for a protein boost
- Sweet potatoes are rich in beta-carotene, an anti-inflammatory nutrient
- Kale is nutrient-dense, helping to reduce inflammation and support immune health

Nutritional Values: Calories: 180, Fat: 7g, Carbs: 27g, Protein: 4g, Sugar: 6g, Sodium: 75 mg, Potassium: 447 mg, Cholesterol: 0 mg

Chapter 7: Lunch Recipes

It's the middle of a bustling day. Between meetings, projects, and the often relentless demands of daily life, lunch can feel like just another task on an endless to-do list. Yet, this quick meal, frequently squeezed between commitments, holds more power than we might think—especially when it comes to reducing inflammation and replenishing our energy.

Imagine walking into your lunch break with a sense of calm anticipation, knowing that you have a delicious meal waiting that will not only satisfy your hunger but also nurture your body. In this chapter, we explore a series of easy, delightful recipes that are designed to be both convenient and beneficial. They are your midday boost, subtly engineered to combat inflammation and boost your well-being without demanding more time than you can spare.

These recipes take familiar favorites and reinvent them with an anti-inflammatory twist. Think vibrant salads rich in omega-3s and antioxidants, wraps filled with colorful, crisp vegetables, and hearty soups that warm and soothe. Each dish is crafted to deliver maximum flavor and health benefits with minimal fuss, aligning with your life's pace without compromising your dietary goals.

Beyond mere sustenance, these lunch recipes are about transforming your relationship with food. They encourage you to pause, even if briefly, and savor the flavors that feed more than just your body. They are a testament to the fact that food can be quick without being rushed, healthy without being restrictive, and indulgent without being detrimental.

Let's redefine the concept of a 'working lunch.' Let this be your invitation to treat your midday meal as a small, sacred ritual—a potent mix of nourishment and pleasure, poised to heal and invigorate. Through these pages, we'll discover that even on the busiest days, lunch can be a respite and a resource, a moment of peace amid the chaos where our dietary choices become our allies in pursuing a vibrant, healthful life.

Kale and Quinoa Power Bowl

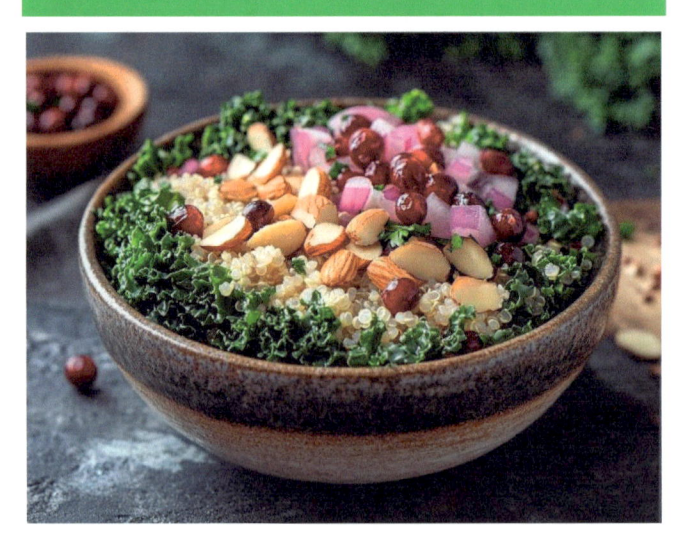

Preparation Time: 15 min
Cooking Time: 20 min
Mode of Cooking: Boiling and Tossing
Servings: 2

Ingredients:
- 1 C. quinoa, rinsed
- 2 C. water
- 1 bunch kale, stems removed and leaves torn
- 1 Tbsp extra virgin olive oil
- 1 tsp apple cider vinegar
- 1 small red onion, thinly sliced
- 1/4 C. dried cranberries
- 1/4 C. slivered almonds, toasted
- 1 tsp grated ginger
- Sea salt and black pepper to taste

Directions:
1. Rinse quinoa thoroughly and boil in water until quinoa is fluffy and water is absorbed
2. In a separate bowl, toss kale with olive oil, vinegar, and seasonings until leaves begin to soften
3. Combine quinoa, kale, onion, cranberries, almonds, and ginger; mix well

Tips:
- Serve warm or chilled for enhanced flavors
- Add a squeeze of lemon juice right before serving to enhance the antioxidant properties
- Consider adding a sprinkle of turmeric for an extra anti-inflammatory boost

Nutritional Values: Calories: 310, Fat: 9g, Carbs: 49g, Protein: 8g, Sugar: 10g, Sodium: 30 mg, Potassium: 450 mg, Cholesterol: 0 mg

CHICKPEA AND AVOCADO GARDEN SALAD

Preparation Time: 10 min
Cooking Time: none
Mode of Cooking: Mixing
Servings: 2

Ingredients:
- 1 C. canned chickpeas, rinsed and drained
- 1 ripe avocado, pitted and diced
- 1/2 C. cherry tomatoes, halved
- 1/4 C. cucumber, diced
- 2 Tbsp red onion, finely chopped
- 2 Tbsp cilantro, chopped
- 1 Tbsp lime juice
- 1 Tbsp extra virgin olive oil
- Salt and pepper to taste
- 1/4 tsp cumin powder

Directions:
1. In a large bowl, combine all ingredients; toss gently to mix
2. Adjust seasoning with salt, pepper, and extra lime juice as per taste

Tips:
- Try replacing lime juice with lemon for a different citrus note
- Adding diced red bell pepper will not only add a splash of color but also boost Vitamin C content

Nutritional Values: Calories: 275, Fat: 15g, Carbs: 30g, Protein: 7g, Sugar: 5g, Sodium: 300 mg, Potassium: 485 mg, Cholesterol: 0 mg

Spinach and Strawberry Crisp Salad

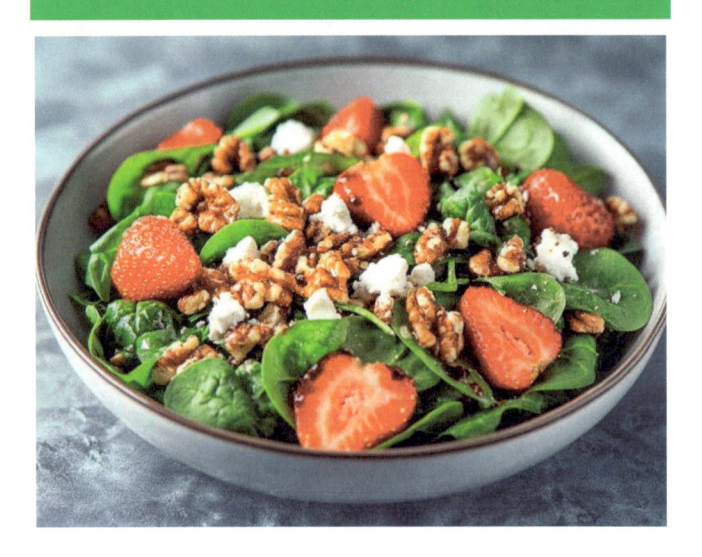

Preparation Time: 10 min
Cooking Time: none
Mode of Cooking: Mixing
Servings: 2
Ingredients:

- 2 C. fresh spinach, washed and dried
- 1 C. strawberries, sliced
- 1/4 C. walnuts, crushed
- 1/4 C. goat cheese, crumbled
- 2 Tbsp balsamic vinegar
- 1 Tbsp honey
- 1 Tbsp extra virgin olive oil
- Salt and black pepper to taste

Directions:

1. Combine balsamic vinegar, honey, olive oil, salt, and pepper in a small bowl and whisk until well blended
2. In a larger bowl, combine spinach, strawberries, walnuts, and goat cheese
3. Drizzle dressing over salad and toss gently to coat

Tips:

- Sprinkle a bit of flaxseed on top for an omega-3 boost
- Chill the salad for about an hour before serving to merge the flavors beautifully

Nutritional Values: Calories: 250, Fat: 18g, Carbs: 20g, Protein: 6g, Sugar: 12g, Sodium: 125 mg, Potassium: 350 mg, Cholesterol: 15 mg

Roasted Beet and Arugula Salad

Preparation Time: 10 min
Cooking Time: 25 min
Mode of Cooking: Roasting and Mixing
Servings: 2
Ingredients:

- 3 medium beets, peeled and cubed
- 2 C. arugula
- 1/4 C. feta cheese, crumbled
- 1/4 C. pistachios, shelled and chopped
- 2 Tbsp olive oil
- 1 Tbsp red wine vinegar
- 1 tsp honey
- Salt and black pepper to taste
- 1/2 tsp dried thyme

Directions:

1. Preheat oven to 375°F (190°C)
2. Toss beets in 1 Tbsp olive oil and roast until tender
3. Whisk together remaining oil, vinegar, honey, thyme, salt, and pepper
4. Combine roasted beets, arugula, feta, and pistachios in a salad bowl and toss with dressing

Tips:

- Roasting the beets can be done in advance to save time
- This salad pairs well with grilled chicken or fish for a complete meal
- Feta can be substituted with goat cheese for a different flavor profile

Nutritional Values: Calories: 290, Fat: 20g, Carbs: 23g, Protein: 7g, Sugar: 16g, Sodium: 320 mg, Potassium: 530 mg, Cholesterol: 25 mg

MEDITERRANEAN LENTIL BOWL

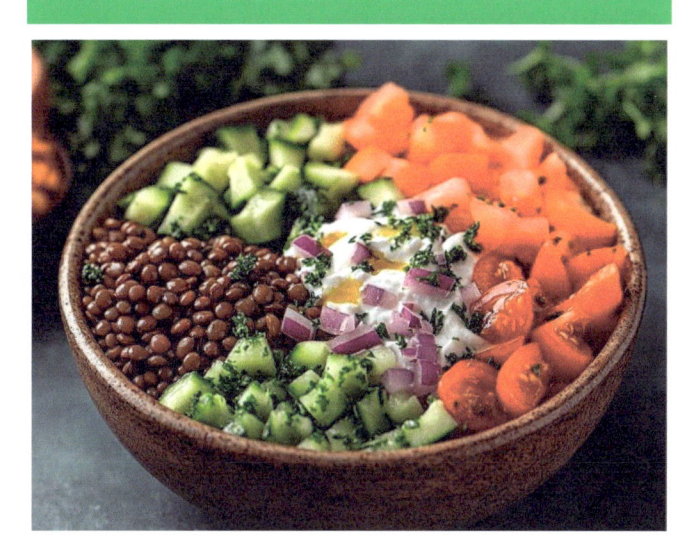

Preparation Time: 15 min
Cooking Time: 25 min
Mode of Cooking: Boiling and Assembling
Servings: 2
Ingredients:

- 1 C. green lentils, rinsed
- 2 C. vegetable broth
- 1/2 C. cherry tomatoes, halved
- 1/2 C. cucumber, diced
- 1/4 C. red onion, thinly sliced
- 1/4 C. kalamata olives, halved
- 2 Tbsp parsley, chopped
- 2 Tbsp lemon juice
- 1 Tbsp extra virgin olive oil
- Salt and pepper to taste
- 1/4 tsp paprika

Directions:

1. Boil lentils in vegetable broth until tender, drain any excess liquid
2. In a large mixing bowl, combine cooked lentils with tomatoes, cucumber, onion, olives, and parsley
3. Dress with lemon juice, olive oil, and season with salt, pepper, and paprika

Tips:

- To add a creamy texture, top with dollops of Greek yogurt
- For an extra antioxidant boost, sprinkle some dried oregano on top before serving

Nutritional Values: Calories: 315, Fat: 9g, Carbs: 45g, Protein: 18g, Sugar: 4g, Sodium: 150 mg, Potassium: 710 mg, Cholesterol: 0 mg

COCONUT CURRY SOUP

Preparation Time: 15 min
Cooking Time: 25 min
Mode of Cooking: Simmering
Servings: 4
Ingredients:

- 1 Tbsp coconut oil
- 1 onion, diced
- 2 Tbsp red curry paste
- 1 bell pepper, sliced
- 1 zucchini, sliced
- 4 cups vegetable broth
- 1 can (14 oz.) coconut milk

- 1 Tbsp fish sauce
- 1 Tbsp brown sugar
- 3 Tbsp lime juice
- Salt to taste
- Fresh cilantro for garnish

Directions:

1. Heat coconut oil in a large pot over medium heat
2. Add onion, sauté until soft
3. Stir in curry paste, cook for 1 min
4. Add bell pepper and zucchini, sauté for another 5 min
5. Pour in vegetable broth and coconut milk, bring to a simmer
6. Add fish sauce, brown sugar, and lime juice, simmer for 15 min
7. Season with salt, garnish with cilantro before serving

Tips:

- Add shredded chicken or tofu for extra protein
- Sprinkle with chili flakes for additional spice
- Coconut milk is rich in anti-inflammatory fatty acids, making it an excellent choice for this soothing soup

Nutritional Values: Calories: 210, Fat: 16g, Carbs: 15g, Protein: 3g, Sugar: 8g, Sodium: 350 mg, Potassium: 430 mg, Cholesterol: 0 mg

GRILLED CHICKEN WRAP

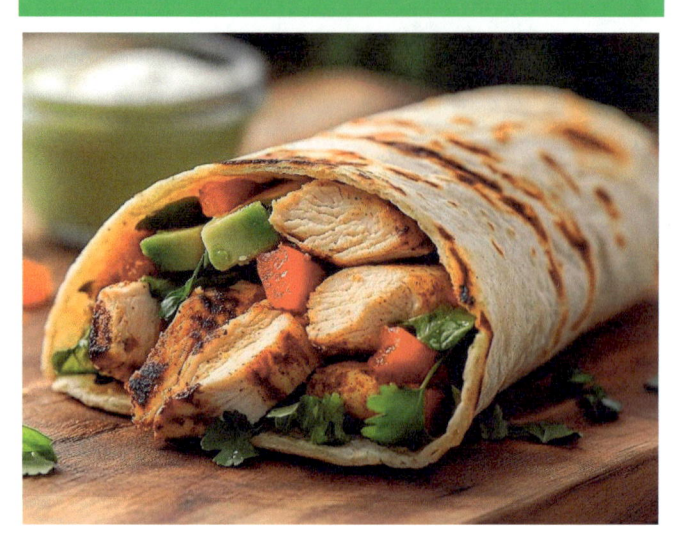

Preparation Time: 20 min
Cooking Time: 10 min
Mode of Cooking: Grilling
Servings: 2
Ingredients:

- 1 large chicken breast
- 2 whole wheat tortillas
- 1 avocado, thinly sliced
- 1 cup mixed greens
- 1/2 red bell pepper, julienned
- 1 Tbsp olive oil
- 1 tsp smoked paprika
- 1/2 tsp garlic powder
- Salt and pepper to taste
- 1 Tbsp fresh lime juice

Directions:

1. Rub chicken breast with olive oil, smoked paprika, garlic powder, salt, and pepper
2. grill on medium heat until cooked through, about 5 min each side
3. let rest for 5 min then slice

4. warm tortillas on the grill for about 1 min each side
5. assemble wraps by placing greens, bell pepper, avocado slices, and chicken on tortillas
6. sprinkle with lime juice, wrap tightly

Tips:

• Use Greek yogurt as a dressing base to add probiotics

• Include a pinch of cayenne for added heat and enhanced metabolism

Nutritional Values: Calories: 365, Fat: 14g, Carbs: 34g, Protein: 26g, Sugar: 3g, Sodium: 200 mg, Potassium: 550 mg, Cholesterol: 70 mg

HUMMUS AND VEGGIE SANDWICH

Preparation Time: 15 min
Cooking Time: none
Mode of Cooking: No cooking
Servings: 2
Ingredients:

- 4 slices whole grain bread
- 1 cup homemade hummus
- 1 cucumber, thinly sliced
- 2 small carrots, shredded
- 1/2 red onion, thinly sliced
- 1/4 cup alfalfa sprouts
- Salt and pepper to taste

Directions:

1. Spread hummus evenly on all bread slices
2. layer cucumber, carrots, red onion, and sprouts over two of the bread slices
3. season with salt and pepper
4. cover with the remaining slices, press down gently to adhere

Tips:

• Swap hummus with guacamole for a twist on flavor and fats

• Add sliced radishes for a peppery crunch

Nutritional Values: Calories: 290, Fat: 9g, Carbs: 42g, Protein: 12g, Sugar: 6g, Sodium: 390 mg, Potassium: 460 mg, Cholesterol: 0 mg

AVOCADO CHICKPEA WRAP

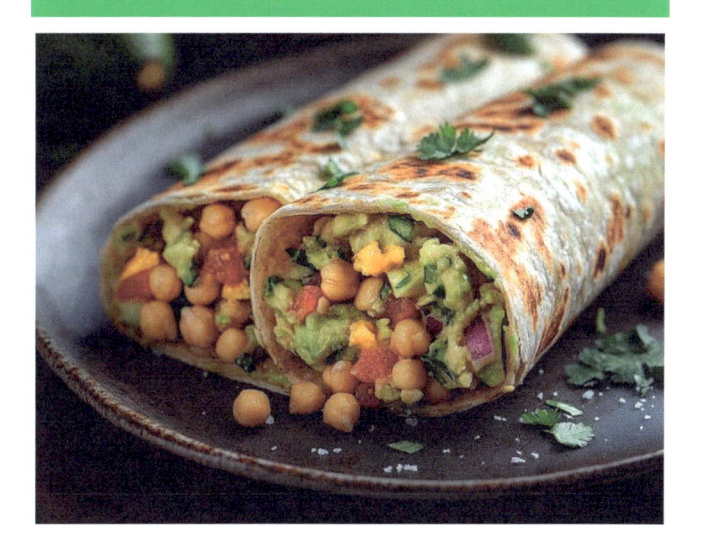

Preparation Time: 10 min
Cooking Time: none
Mode of Cooking: No Cooking
Servings: 2
Ingredients:

- 2 whole wheat tortillas
- 1 ripe avocado, mashed
- 1 cup canned chickpeas, rinsed and mashed
- 1 small tomato, diced
- 1/4 cup red onion, finely diced
- 2 Tbsp cilantro, chopped
- 1 Tbsp lemon juice
- Salt and pepper to taste

Directions:

1. Combine avocado, chickpeas, tomato, red onion, cilantro, lemon juice, salt, and pepper in a bowl
2. mash until well mixed but still chunky
3. spread mixture over tortillas
4. roll tightly

Tips:

- Enhance flavor with a sprinkle of cumin
- Incorporate chopped spinach for extra iron and vitamin K

Nutritional Values: Calories: 400, Fat: 20g, Carbs: 45g, Protein: 11g, Sugar: 5g, Sodium: 200 mg, Potassium: 420 mg, Cholesterol: 0 mg

TURKEY AND SPINACH SANDWICH

Preparation Time: 15 min
Cooking Time: none
Mode of Cooking: No Cooking
Servings: 2
Ingredients:

- 4 slices rye bread
- 4 oz roasted turkey breast, thinly sliced
- 1 cup spinach leaves
- 2 Tbsp mustard
- 1/4 red onion, thinly sliced
- 1 Tbsp mayo, optional

Directions:

1. Spread mustard (and mayo, if using) on bread slices
2. layer turkey, spinach, and onion slices on two bread slices
3. cover with the remaining bread slices

Tips:

- Try adding slices of pear for a sweet crunch
- Use whole grain mustard for extra texture and flavor

Nutritional Values: Calories: 310, Fat: 9g, Carbs: 35g, Protein: 25g, Sugar: 4g, Sodium: 870 mg, Potassium: 310 mg, Cholesterol: 55 mg

Chapter 8: Dinner Recipes

Evening meals hold a special place in our lives; they are not just about refueling after a long day, but about unwinding, sharing moments with family, and transitioning gracefully towards a restful night. That's why the dinner recipes in this chapter are designed to soothe inflammation and foster a sense of peace and well-being, without spending hours in the kitchen.

Imagine this: The setting sun paints your kitchen golden as you begin to prepare a meal that's as nurturing to your body as it is delightful to your taste buds. Dinner, in many ways, acts as a gentle closure to the day's hustle and can significantly influence how peacefully we sleep and how rejuvenated we feel upon waking. With this in mind, each recipe here has been crafted to balance ease of preparation with nutritional benefit, ensuring that you can relax and enjoy the process of cooking as much as eating.

In this chapter, you will find dishes rich in omega-3 fatty acids from sources like succulent salmon or creamy avocados, ideal for their anti-inflammatory prowess. Moreover, vibrant vegetables and whole grains feature prominently, providing both texture and a treasure trove of antioxidants. From a simple, hearty stew that allows the slow cooker to do most of the work, to a quick, aromatic stir-fry that encapsulates bold flavors within minutes, there's something for every palate and schedule.

Beyond the recipes themselves, consider this chapter a guide on how to end your day nutritionally empowered. For those evenings when time slips through your fingers, you'll pick up strategies for quick, wholesome dinners that don't sacrifice flavor or health benefits. On nights when you find a few extra moments, dive into a recipe that's slightly more elaborate, a small adventure in your kitchen that celebrates your achievements of the day.

Ultimately, these dinner recipes are designed not just to minimize inflammation, but to maximize joy and satisfaction in your evening meal. As we settle down for dinner, let's embrace the power of nourishing food to heal and harmonize our bodies and minds, ensuring that every night ends on a delicious, peaceful note.

Herb-Marinated Grilled Salmon

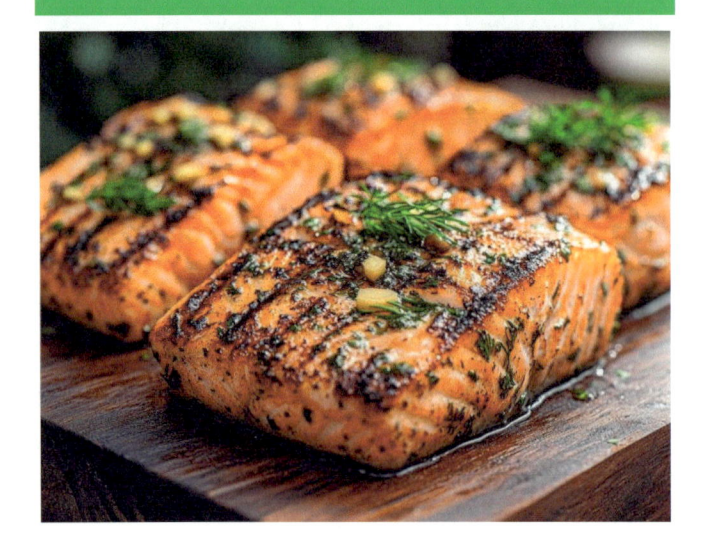

Preparation Time: 15 min
Cooking Time: 20 min
Mode of Cooking: Grilling
Servings: 4
Ingredients:
- 4 salmon fillets, about 6 oz. each
- 3 Tbsp extra virgin olive oil
- 2 garlic cloves, minced
- 2 Tbsp fresh dill, chopped
- 2 Tbsp fresh parsley, chopped
- 1 Tbsp fresh lemon juice
- Salt and pepper to taste

Directions:
1. Combine olive oil, garlic, dill, parsley, lemon juice, salt, and pepper in a bowl
2. Place salmon fillets in a shallow dish and pour marinade over them, ensuring each fillet is well coated
3. Marinate in the refrigerator for at least 10 min before grilling
4. Preheat grill to medium-high heat (about 450°F (232°C))
5. Grill salmon on each side for about 10 min until cooked through and flaky

Tips:
- Use fresh herbs for the best flavor and nutrient content
- Grill over indirect heat to prevent drying out the salmon
- Drizzle with a bit of extra virgin olive oil before serving to enhance flavor

Nutritional Values: Calories: 280, Fat: 18g, Carbs: 0g, Protein: 23g, Sugar: 0g, Sodium: 75mg, Potassium: 500mg, Cholesterol: 60mg

Lemon Garlic Chicken Breasts

Preparation Time: 10 min
Cooking Time: 30 min
Mode of Cooking: Baking
Servings: 4
Ingredients:
- 4 boneless, skinless chicken breasts
- 4 cloves garlic, minced
- 3 Tbsp olive oil
- 1 Tbsp lemon zest
- 2 Tbsp lemon juice
- 1 tsp dried oregano
- Salt and pepper to taste

Directions:
1. Mix garlic, olive oil, lemon zest, lemon juice, oregano, salt, and pepper in a bowl to create marinade
2. Place chicken breasts in a baking dish and cover with marinade, marinate for at least 15 min in the refrigerator
3. Preheat oven to 375°F (190°C)

4. Bake chicken for 25-30 min until fully cooked and juices run clear

Tips:

• To keep chicken moist, cover the baking dish with aluminum foil during the first 20 min of baking

• Serve with a side of steamed vegetables to make a balanced meal

• Lemon zest adds a refreshing flavor and boosts antioxidant content

Nutritional Values: Calories: 225, Fat: 10g, Carbs: 3g, Protein: 30g, Sugar: 1g, Sodium: 65mg, Potassium: 290mg, Cholesterol: 80mg

SPICED TOFU STIR-FRY

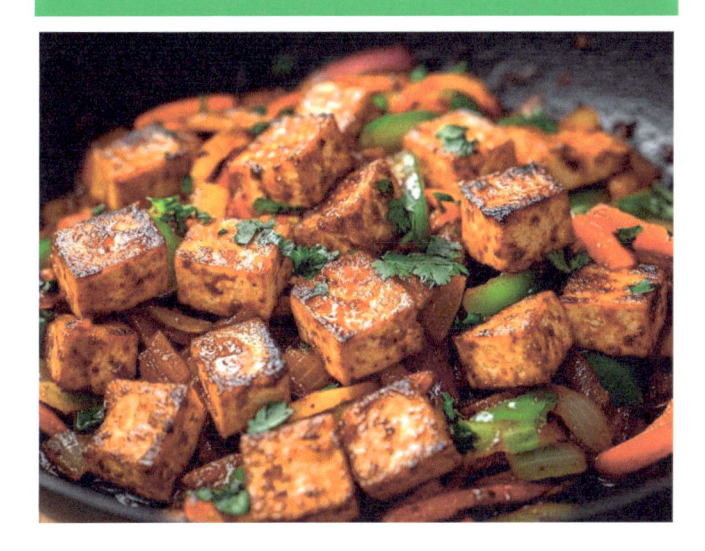

Preparation Time: 15 min
Cooking Time: 10 min
Mode of Cooking: Stir-Frying
Servings: 4
Ingredients:

• 14 oz. firm tofu, drained and cubed
• 2 Tbsp sesame oil
• 1 red bell pepper, sliced
• 1 green bell pepper, sliced
• 1 onion, thinly sliced
• 2 Tbsp soy sauce
• 1 Tbsp minced ginger
• 1 tsp ground turmeric
• 1 tsp ground cumin

Directions:

1. Heat sesame oil in a large skillet or wok over medium-high heat
2. Add onion and bell peppers and stir-fry for about 5 min until tender
3. Add cubed tofu, soy sauce, ginger, turmeric, and cumin
4. Cook for an additional 5 min, stirring frequently to prevent sticking and to ensure that tofu is evenly coated with spices

Tips:

• Add a splash of water or vegetable broth if the stir-fry appears too dry or begins to stick

• Garnish with fresh cilantro or scallions for added flavor and a vibrant presentation

• Turmeric and ginger are powerful anti-inflammatory agents

Nutritional Values: Calories: 180, Fat: 12g, Carbs: 8g, Protein: 12g, Sugar: 3g, Sodium: 530mg, Potassium: 200mg, Cholesterol: 0mg

GINGER-LIME SHRIMP

Preparation Time: 10 min
Cooking Time: 8 min
Mode of Cooking: Sautéing
Servings: 4
Ingredients:

• 1 lb. shrimp, peeled and deveined
• 2 Tbsp extra virgin olive oil

- 1 Tbsp lime zest
- 3 Tbsp lime juice
- 1 Tbsp minced ginger
- 1 clove garlic, minced
- 1/4 tsp red pepper flakes
- Salt to taste

Directions:

1. Mix lime zest, lime juice, ginger, garlic, red pepper flakes, and salt together to form a marinade
2. Toss the shrimp in the marinade and let sit for about 10 min
3. Heat olive oil in a skillet over medium-high heat
4. Sauté shrimp for about 4 min per side or until pink and cooked through

Tips:

- Do not overcook the shrimp to avoid a rubbery texture
- Pair with a side of quinoa for a complete meal rich in protein and fiber
- The combination of ginger and lime not only enhances flavor but also offers significant anti-inflammatory benefits

Nutritional Values: Calories: 160, Fat: 8g, Carbs: 3g, Protein: 20g, Sugar: 0g, Sodium: 190mg, Potassium: 300mg, Cholesterol: 150mg

BALSAMIC GLAZED PORK CHOPS

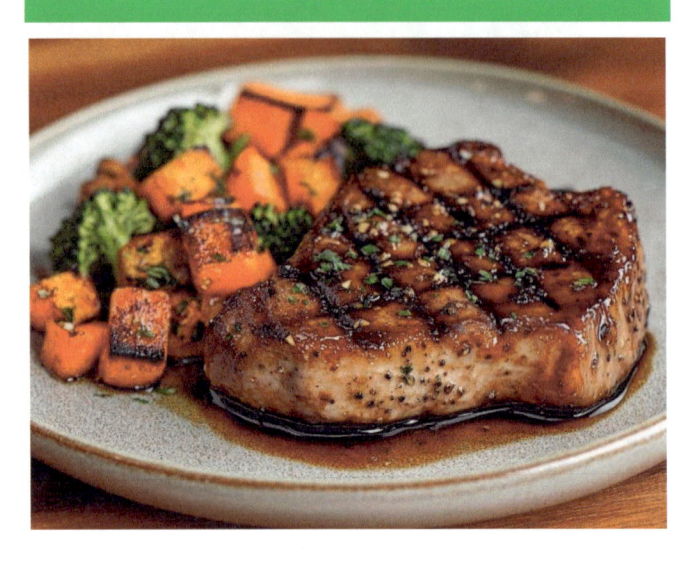

Preparation Time: 20 min
Cooking Time: 15 min
Mode of Cooking: Pan-Searing
Servings: 4
Ingredients:

- 4 pork chops, about 1-inch thick
- 2 Tbsp balsamic vinegar
- 1 Tbsp honey
- 2 cloves garlic, minced
- 2 Tbsp extra virgin olive oil
- 1 tsp dried rosemary
- Salt and pepper to taste

Directions:

1. Combine balsamic vinegar, honey, garlic, olive oil, rosemary, salt, and pepper in a bowl to create glaze
2. Coat pork chops in the glaze and set aside to marinate for 15 min
3. Heat a skillet over medium-high heat and sear each pork chop for about 7 min on each side or until cooked to desired doneness

Tips:

- Allow meat to rest for 5 min before serving to reabsorb juices
- Serve with a side of roasted vegetables tossed in olive oil and herbs
- Honey in the balsamic glaze helps to caramelize the surface of the pork chops, enhancing their natural flavors and adding anti-inflammatory properties

Nutritional Values: Calories: 300, Fat: 16g, Carbs: 5g, Protein: 30g, Sugar: 4g, Sodium: 70mg, Potassium: 500mg, Cholesterol: 90mg

ROASTED CAULIFLOWER STEAKS WITH TURMERIC AND GARLIC

Preparation Time: 15 min
Cooking Time: 25 min
Mode of Cooking: Roasting
Servings: 4
Ingredients:

- 1 large head cauliflower, sliced into 4 steaks
- 3 Tbsp olive oil
- 2 tsp turmeric
- 3 cloves garlic, minced
- Salt and pepper to taste
- Fresh parsley, chopped for garnish

Directions:

1. Preheat oven to 400°F (200°C)
2. Place cauliflower steaks on a baking sheet
3. In a small bowl, mix olive oil, turmeric, and minced garlic
4. Brush mixture over both sides of each cauliflower steak
5. Season with salt and pepper
6. Roast in the oven for about 25 min, flipping halfway through until golden and tender
7. Garnish with fresh parsley before serving

Tips:

- Serve with a side of mixed greens for an enhanced meal
- Cauliflower and turmeric are powerful anti-inflammatory agents, aiding in reducing inflammation and boosting antioxidant intake

Nutritional Values: Calories: 164, Fat: 14g, Carbs: 10g, Protein: 3g, Sugar: 3g, Sodium: 45 mg, Potassium: 320 mg, Cholesterol: 0 mg

ZUCCHINI NOODLES WITH AVOCADO PESTO

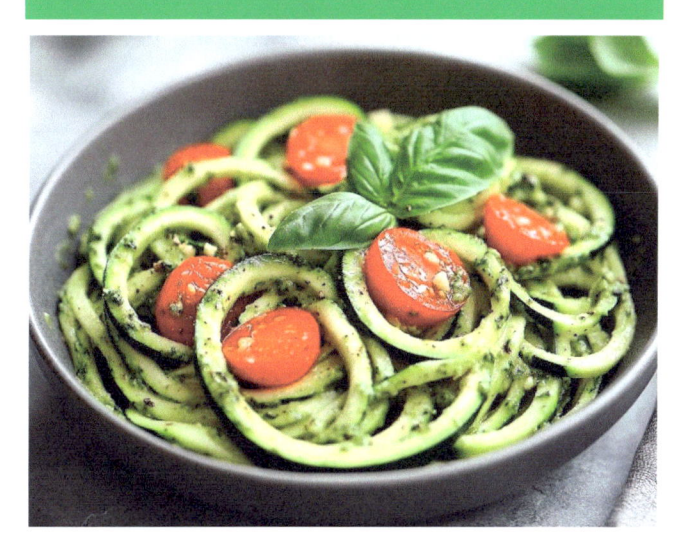

Preparation Time: 10 min
Cooking Time: none
Mode of Cooking: Raw
Servings: 2
Ingredients:

- 3 zucchinis, spiralized into noodles
- 1 ripe avocado
- 1/2 cup fresh basil leaves
- 1/4 cup pine nuts

- 2 cloves garlic
- 2 Tbsp lemon juice
- Salt and pepper to taste
- Cherry tomatoes for garnish

Directions:

1. Combine avocado, basil, pine nuts, garlic, and lemon juice in a blender or food processor until smooth
2. Season with salt and pepper
3. Toss zucchini noodles with avocado pesto until well coated
4. Serve topped with cherry tomatoes

Tips:

- Add a sprinkle of nutritional yeast for a cheesy flavor without the dairy
- Avocado and pine nuts are rich in healthy fats and antioxidants, helping diminish inflammation

Nutritional Values: Calories: 421, Fat: 31g, Carbs: 35g, Protein: 8g, Sugar: 10g, Sodium: 42 mg, Potassium: 1432 mg, Cholesterol: 0 mg

CAULIFLOWER MAC AND CHEESE

Preparation Time: 15 min
Cooking Time: 25 min
Mode of Cooking: Baking
Servings: 4
Ingredients:

- 1 large cauliflower head, cut into florets
- 2 Tbsp unsalted butter
- 2 Tbsp spelt flour
- 2 cups unsweetened almond milk
- 1/2 tsp garlic powder
- 1/2 tsp mustard powder
- 1 cup grated cheddar cheese, reduced-fat
- Salt and pepper to taste

Directions:

1. Steam cauliflower until tender
2. Melt butter in a saucepan, whisk in flour to form a roux
3. Gradually add almond milk, stirring continuously until thickened
4. Mix in garlic powder, mustard powder, and cheese until melted
5. Season with salt and pepper to taste
6. Combine cheese sauce with cauliflower and transfer to a baking dish
7. Bake at 350°F (175°C) until bubbly and lightly browned

Tips:

- Swap regular cheese with nutritional yeast for a vegan option with a cheese-like flavor and added vitamins
- Incorporate a pinch of turmeric in the cheese sauce for extra anti-inflammatory benefits
- Serve with a side of green salad to incorporate more anti-inflammatory ingredients

Nutritional Values: Calories: 270, Fat: 16g, Carbs: 18g, Protein: 12g, Sugar: 5g, Sodium: 340 mg, Potassium: 470 mg, Cholesterol: 30 mg

Lentil Bolognese

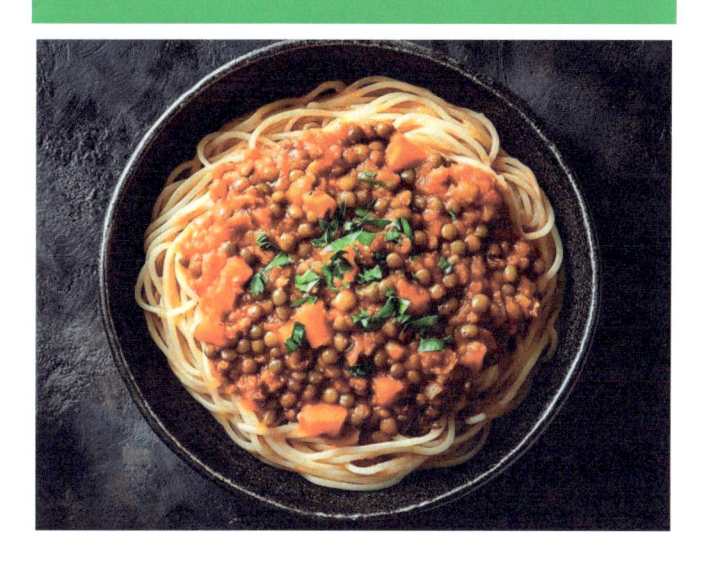

Preparation Time: 10 min
Cooking Time: 30 min
Mode of Cooking: Simmering
Servings: 5
Ingredients:

- 1 cup brown lentils, rinsed
- 1 onion, chopped
- 2 garlic cloves, minced
- 1 carrot, diced
- 1 celery stalk, diced
- 3 cups crushed tomatoes
- 1 Tbsp olive oil
- 1 tsp dried basil
- 1 tsp dried oregano
- Salt and pepper to taste
- Fresh basil for garnish

Directions:

1. Heat olive oil in a pan, saute onion, garlic, carrot, and celery until soft
2. Add lentils and crushed tomatoes, bring to a simmer
3. Add basil, oregano, salt, and pepper and cook until lentils are tender
4. Serve over cooked whole wheat spaghetti or zucchini noodles
5. Garnish with fresh basil

Tips:

- Adding a splash of balsamic vinegar at the end of cooking can boost flavor and provide antioxidants
- Consider using fire-roasted tomatoes for a slightly smoky flavor
- This sauce can be made in large batches and frozen for future quick and healthy meals

Nutritional Values: Calories: 230, Fat: 3g, Carbs: 40g, Protein: 12g, Sugar: 6g, Sodium: 20 mg, Potassium: 705 mg, Cholesterol: 0 mg

Chicken and Veggie Casserole

Preparation Time: 15 min
Cooking Time: 40 min
Mode of Cooking: Baking
Servings: 6
Ingredients:

- 1 lb chicken breast, diced
- 1 cup broccoli florets
- 1 cup bell peppers, sliced
- 1 cup carrots, sliced
- 1 onion, chopped
- 2 garlic cloves, minced
- 1 Tbsp olive oil
- 1 tsp Italian seasoning
- 1/2 cup low-fat Greek yogurt
- 1/2 cup grated Parmesan cheese
- Salt and pepper to taste

Directions:

1. Preheat oven to 375°F (190°C)

2. In a large skillet, heat olive oil and saute garlic and onion until translucent
3. Add chicken and cook until no longer pink
4. Mix in broccoli, bell peppers, and carrots and cook for 5 min
5. Stir in Greek yogurt, Parmesan, Italian seasoning, salt, and pepper
6. Transfer mixture to a baking dish and bake until vegetables are tender and top is slightly browned

Tips:

- Using Greek yogurt instead of cream reduces fat content and adds protein and probiotics
- Experiment with different vegetable combinations like zucchini or spinach to keep meals exciting and nutritionally varied
- Sprinkle almond slices on top before baking for added crunch and healthy fats

Nutritional Values: Calories: 250, Fat: 7g, Carbs: 15g, Protein: 33g, Sugar: 5g, Sodium: 220 mg, Potassium: 500 mg, Cholesterol: 65 mg

Chapter 9: Snacks and Small Bites

It's mid-afternoon and you find yourself searching the kitchen for something to nibble on. Let's be honest, the allure of unhealthy snacks is difficult to resist, especially during a busy day. But imagine having a selection of delightful treats that are not only satisfying to your taste buds but also nourishing to your body. Welcome to the heart of healthy snacking—where every bite counts not just to quell your hunger but to combat inflammation and boost your wellbeing.

In this chapter on Snacks and Small Bites, we'll explore how the simplicity of a snack can be your secret weapon in maintaining an anti-inflammatory lifestyle. The key lies in choosing ingredients that are rich in nutrients, low in processed sugars, and abundant in natural flavors—foods that make you feel good both inside and out.

Think about the ease of assembling a vibrant plate of hummus paired with crisp, colorful vegetables, or the rustic charm of homemade nut bars, rich with seeds and subtle sweetness. These snacks are designed not only to be quick and convenient but also to provide a powerful punch of anti-inflammatory benefits. Each recipe has been crafted to ensure that you're not only satiated but also taking strides toward a healthier, more vibrant self.

Our goal here is not to add another layer of complexity to your already bustling day but to show you how effortlessly these small bites can integrate into your lifestyle. Whether you find comfort in the crunch of a fresh apple with almond butter or the zesty zing of a mango salsa, these snacks are about celebrating the natural goodness of whole foods without compromising on taste.

By the end of this chapter, you'll have a new repertoire of snacks that are as easy to prepare as they are beneficial for your health. So, let's embark on this snacking adventure together, where each small bite is a step towards a healthier you. Embrace this opportunity to transform your snacking habits into a joyful, nourishing practice that supports your body's needs and your soul's cravings.

Beetroot and Apple Juice

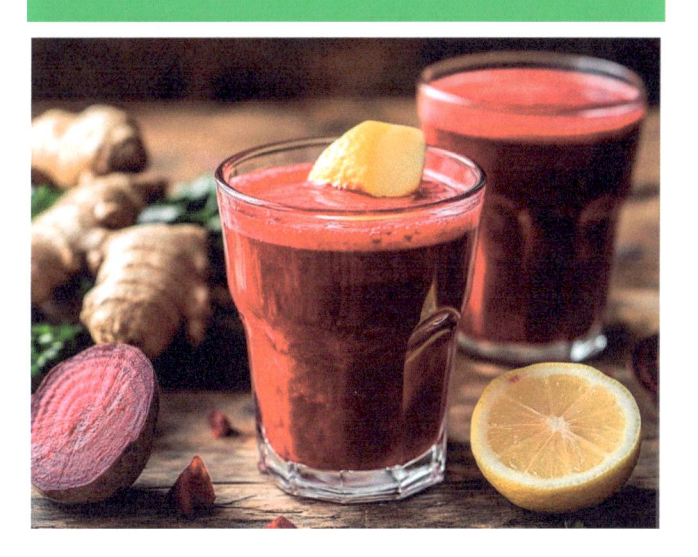

Preparation Time: 5 min
Cooking Time: none
Mode of Cooking: Blending
Servings: 2

Ingredients:
- 2 medium beetroots, peeled and chopped
- 1 large apple, cored and sliced
- 1 inch fresh ginger, peeled
- 1/2 lemon, juiced
- 1 cup cold water
- 5 ice cubes

Directions:
1. Add all ingredients to a high-powered blender
2. Blend on high until smooth
3. Strain if desired and serve immediately

Tips:
- Add a pinch of ground cinnamon for a warm spice note
- Use a tart apple variety like Granny Smith for a vibrant flavor contrast
- Beetroot is rich in nitrates and betalains, which are known for their anti-inflammatory properties

Nutritional Values: Calories: 95, Fat: 0.3g, Carbs: 23g, Protein: 1.5g, Sugar: 17g, Sodium: 76 mg, Potassium: 400 mg, Cholesterol: 0 mg

CARROT GINGER SMOOTHIE

Preparation Time: 7 min
Cooking Time: none
Mode of Cooking: Blending
Servings: 2

Ingredients:
- 3 large carrots, peeled and chopped
- 1 inch ginger, peeled
- 1/2 frozen banana
- 1 Tbsp flaxseed meal
- 2 cups unsweetened almond milk
- 1 tsp vanilla extract
- Dash of cinnamon

Directions:
1. Combine carrots, ginger, banana, flaxseed meal, almond milk, vanilla extract, and cinnamon in a blender
2. Blend until smooth
3. Serve chilled

Tips:
- Include a tablespoon of chia seeds to boost omega-3 fatty acid intake
- Ginger is excellent for reducing inflammation and supporting digestive health
- Carrots are a great source of beta-carotene, which is an antioxidant that helps in fighting inflammation

Nutritional Values: Calories: 130, Fat: 4.5g, Carbs: 21g, Protein: 3g, Sugar: 10g, Sodium: 180 mg, Potassium: 750 mg, Cholesterol: 0 mg

GREEN APPLE KALE JUICE

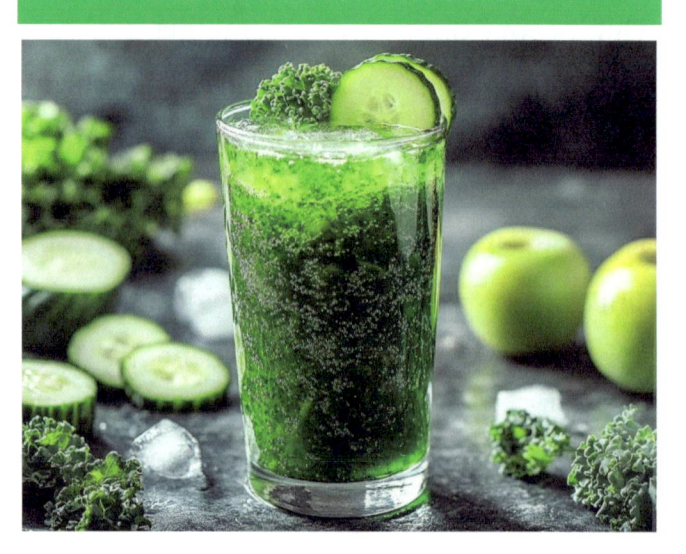

Preparation Time: 8 min
Cooking Time: none

Mode of Cooking: Juicing

Servings: 2

Ingredients:

- 2 green apples, cored and sliced
- 4 large kale leaves
- 1 cucumber, sliced
- 1/2 lime, juiced
- 1/2 cup fresh parsley leaves
- 1 cup water
- 6 ice cubes

Directions:

1. Place all the ingredients except ice cubes into a juicer
2. Juice thoroughly
3. Stir in ice cubes and serve immediately

Tips:

- Adding a handful of mint can enhance the freshness
- Kale and parsley are packed with antioxidants which help in reducing inflammation
- Green apple adds a tartness that balances the bitter notes of kale

Nutritional Values: Calories: 110, Fat: 0.6g, Carbs: 25g, Protein: 3g, Sugar: 14g, Sodium: 30 mg, Potassium: 450 mg, Cholesterol: 0 mg

PINEAPPLE TURMERIC JUICE

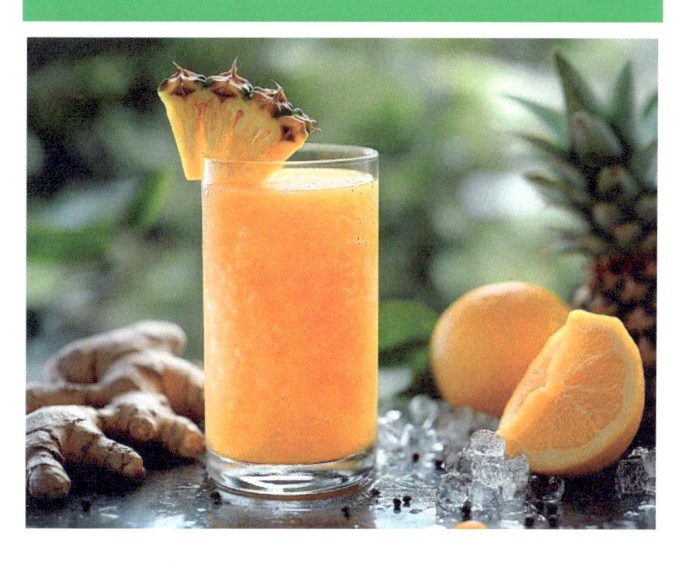

Preparation Time: 6 min

Cooking Time: none

Mode of Cooking: Juicing

Servings: 2

Ingredients:

- 1/2 pineapple, peeled and cored
- 1 inch turmeric root
- 1 inch ginger root
- 1 orange, peeled
- 1/2 lemon, juiced
- 1 cup water
- 5 ice cubes

Directions:

1. Juice pineapple, turmeric root, ginger root, and orange together
2. Pour into glasses
3. Add lemon juice and water
4. Stir in ice cubes and serve immediately

Tips:

- Incorporating a dash of black pepper enhances the absorption of turmeric

- Pineapple contains bromelain, which is known for its anti-inflammatory and digestive benefits
- Turmeric and ginger are renowned for their anti-inflammatory properties

Nutritional Values: Calories: 120, Fat: 0.5g, Carbs: 30g, Protein: 1g, Sugar: 22g, Sodium: 5 mg, Potassium: 490 mg, Cholesterol: 0 mg

BERRY ANTIOXIDANT SMOOTHIE

Preparation Time: 10 min
Cooking Time: none
Mode of Cooking: Blending
Servings: 2
Ingredients:
- 1 cup frozen mixed berries (blueberries, strawberries, raspberries)
- 1 cup spinach leaves
- 1 cup unsweetened coconut water
- 1 Tbsp honey
- 1 Tbsp almond butter
- 1/2 tsp ground turmeric
- 1/2 cup Greek yogurt

Directions:
1. Combine all ingredients in a blender
2. Blend on high until creamy and smooth
3. Serve immediately

Tips:
- Adding a scoop of protein powder can make this a more filling snack
- Berries and turmeric are powerful antioxidants with strong anti-inflammatory effects
- Greek yogurt adds a creamy texture and probiotics

Nutritional Values: Calories: 180, Fat: 5g, Carbs: 28g, Protein: 8g, Sugar: 18g, Sodium: 60 mg, Potassium: 355 mg, Cholesterol: 10 mg

ALMOND COCONUT ENERGY BALLS

Preparation Time: 15 min
Cooking Time: none
Mode of Cooking: No Cooking
Servings: 10
Ingredients:
- 1 cup raw almonds
- ½ cup unsweetened shredded coconut
- ¼ cup chopped dates
- 3 Tbsp raw honey
- 1 tsp vanilla extract
- ¼ tsp sea salt

Directions:
1. Combine almonds, shredded coconut, and dates in a food processor and blend until finely chopped
2. Add honey, vanilla extract, and sea salt to the mixture and process until a sticky dough forms
3. Roll the mixture into small balls, approximately 1-inch in diameter
4. Place on a baking sheet lined with parchment paper and refrigerate until firm

Tips:

- Roll balls in extra shredded coconut or cocoa powder for an added flavor dimension
- Almonds provide a good source of anti-inflammatory Omega-3s
- Refrigerate in an airtight container to preserve freshness

Nutritional Values: Calories: 120, Fat: 9g, Carbs: 8g, Protein: 3g, Sugar: 5g, Sodium: 60mg, Potassium: 125mg, Cholesterol: 0mg

TURMERIC CASHEW BITES

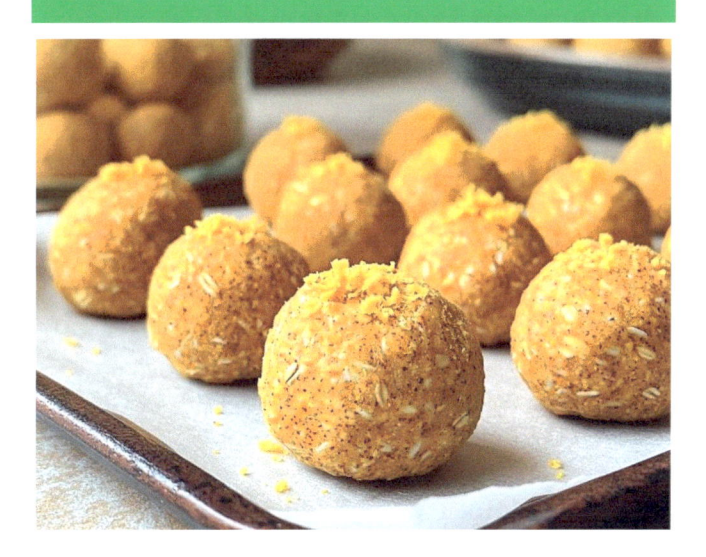

Preparation Time: 20 min
Cooking Time: none
Mode of Cooking: No Cooking
Servings: 8
Ingredients:

- 1 cup cashews
- ½ cup rolled oats
- 2 Tbsp ground flaxseed
- 1 Tbsp turmeric powder
- ¼ cup honey
- 1 tsp lemon zest
- ¼ tsp black pepper
- ¼ tsp salt

Directions:

1. Grind cashews and oats in a food processor until coarse
2. Add flaxseed, turmeric, honey, lemon zest, black pepper, and salt to the processor and blend until sticky
3. Form the mixture into bite-sized balls about 1-inch in diameter
4. Refrigerate on a parchment-lined baking sheet until hardened

Tips:

- Experiment with adding a pinch of cinnamon or ginger for extra flair
- Turmeric and black pepper together enhance anti-inflammatory benefits
- Store in a cool, dry place

Nutritional Values: Calories: 150, Fat: 9g, Carbs: 15g, Protein: 4g, Sugar: 7g, Sodium: 75mg, Potassium: 200mg, Cholesterol: 0mg

DATE AND WALNUT BARS

Preparation Time: 25 min
Cooking Time: none
Mode of Cooking: No Cooking
Servings: 12
Ingredients:

- 1 cup walnuts
- 1 cup dates, pitted and chopped
- ½ cup dried apricots, chopped
- ¼ cup sesame seeds
- 2 Tbsp coconut oil
- 1 Tbsp chia seeds
- 1 tsp orange zest
- Pinch of sea salt

Directions:

1. Process walnuts, dates, and apricots in a food processor until well combined and finely chopped
2. Add sesame seeds, coconut oil, chia seeds, orange zest, and sea salt to the mixture and process until the dough comes together
3. Press the dough into a lined square baking dish and refrigerate until set
4. Cut into bars

Tips:

- Add a sprinkle of hemp seeds before refrigerating for added texture and nutrition
- Walnuts and chia seeds provide essential fatty acids that help combat inflammation
- Wrap individually for quick grab-and-go snacks

Nutritional Values: Calories: 130, Fat: 8g, Carbs: 15g, Protein: 3g, Sugar: 10g, Sodium: 25mg, Potassium: 170mg, Cholesterol: 0mg

CHIA SEED ENERGY BITES

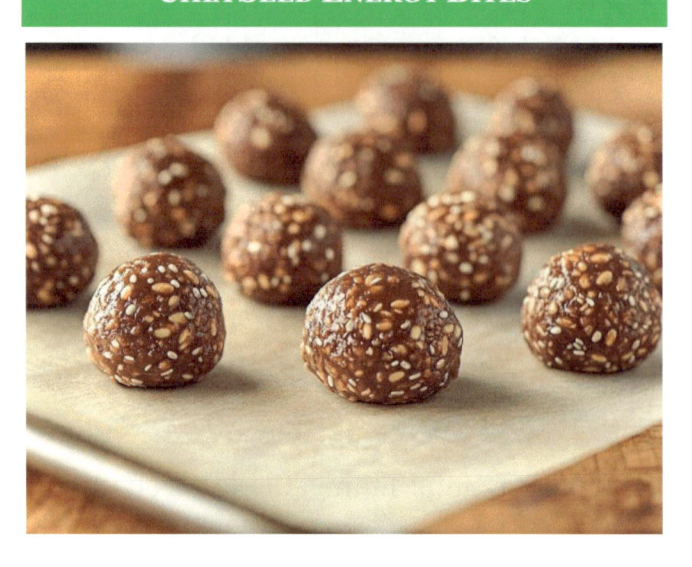

Preparation Time: 15 min
Cooking Time: none
Mode of Cooking: No Cooking
Servings: 12
Ingredients:

- 1 cup oats
- ½ cup chia seeds
- ½ cup almond butter
- ¼ cup honey
- ½ tsp cinnamon
- ¼ tsp vanilla extract

Directions:

1. Mix oats, chia seeds, almond butter, honey, cinnamon, and vanilla extract in a bowl until well incorporated
2. Form the mixture into small balls, about 1-inch in diameter
3. Refrigerate on a tray lined with parchment paper until firm

Tips:

- Try mixing in a few mini dark chocolate chips for a sweet twist

- Chia seeds are rich in antioxidants and provide a crunchy texture to these bites
- Store in a sealed container in the fridge for freshness

Nutritional Values: Calories: 140, Fat: 8g, Carbs: 12g, Protein: 5g, Sugar: 6g, Sodium: 5mg, Potassium: 150mg, Cholesterol: 0mg

PUMPKIN SPICE PROTEIN BALLS

Preparation Time: 18 min
Cooking Time: none
Mode of Cooking: No Cooking
Servings: 10
Ingredients:
- 1 cup pumpkin puree
- ¾ cup oat flour
- ½ cup vanilla protein powder
- ¼ cup almond butter
- 3 Tbsp maple syrup
- 1 tsp pumpkin pie spice
- ¼ tsp salt

Directions:

1. Stir together all ingredients in a large bowl until thoroughly combined
2. Shape the mixture into 1-inch balls
3. Chill on a parchment paper-lined tray in the refrigerator until set

Tips:
- Sprinkle with ground nutmeg or cinnamon before serving for enhanced flavor
- Pumpkin puree is a great source of vitamins and anti-inflammatory benefits
- Perfect as a post-workout snack thanks to the added protein

Nutritional Values: Calories: 100, Fat: 4g, Carbs: 12g, Protein: 6g, Sugar: 4g, Sodium: 55mg, Potassium: 125mg, Cholesterol: 0mg

Chapter 10: Desserts and Treats

Embracing a healthier lifestyle doesn't mean you have to say goodbye to the sweeter things in life. Quite the opposite, actually! In this chapter, we delve into the delicious world of desserts and treats that not only satisfy your sweet tooth but also help combat inflammation and contribute to your overall well-being.

Picture this: It's a quiet evening, and you're craving something sweet after a healthy dinner. Instead of reaching for that usual store-bought ice cream or those pre-packaged cookies loaded with refined sugars and unhealthy fats, you find yourself whipping up a blueberry sorbet laced with anti-inflammatory goodness or a slice of ginger-spiced pumpkin pie that fills your kitchen with enchanting aromas.

This isn't about depriving yourself or sticking to rigid, flavorless dieting rules. On the contrary, it's about reinventing the treats you love with ingredients that love you back. In this chapter, you'll discover how typical inflammatory villains like processed sugar and certain fats can be substituted with natural sweeteners and healthy oils and nuts. These switches not only keep the flavors rich and satisfying but also serve your body's needs for combating inflammation.

Moreover, the dessert recipes featured here are quick to assemble and require minimal ingredients. They are perfect for busy weeknights when you need a simple yet comforting snack, or for impressing guests at your next dinner party without spending all day in the kitchen.

From creamy avocado chocolate mousse to tangy cherry almond tarts, each recipe is a testament to how small, thoughtful changes in your diet can bring about significant health benefits. Not only do these desserts help reduce inflammation, but they also offer vitamins, antioxidants, and minerals crucial for health optimization and stress reduction.

So, let's turn the page and start this sweet adventure, where indulgence meets wellness, proving that you can indeed have your cake and eat it too—without the guilt and with all the health benefits.

Mango Coconut Sorbet

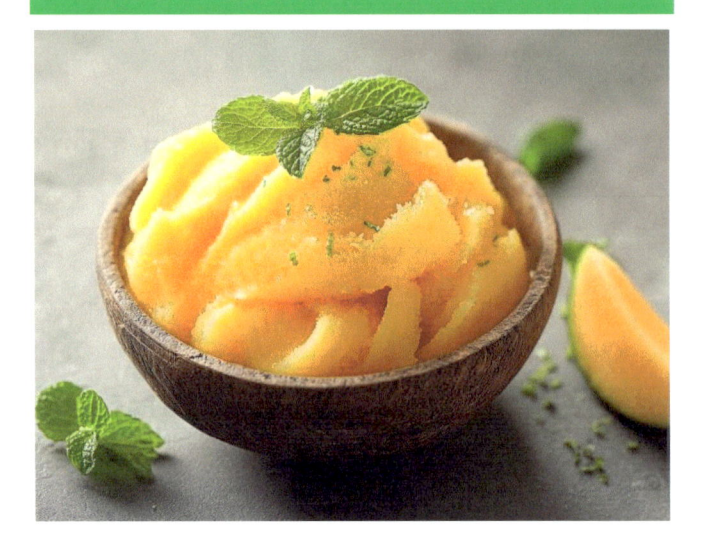

Preparation Time: 15 min
Cooking Time: none
Mode of Cooking: Freezing
Servings: 4

Ingredients:
- 2 ripe mangoes, peeled and cubed
- 1 C. coconut milk
- juice of 1 lime
- 1 Tbsp honey
- 1 tsp fresh ginger, grated

Directions:
1. Blend mangoes, coconut milk, lime juice, honey, and ginger until smooth
2. Pour into a shallow dish
3. Freeze until solid, breaking up and stirring every 30 min.

Tips:
- Sorbet can be blended again before serving for a smoother texture
- Ginger enhances the anti-inflammatory benefits

Nutritional Values: Calories: 180, Fat: 11g, Carbs: 22g, Protein: 1g, Sugar: 20g, Sodium: 15 mg, Potassium: 250 mg, Cholesterol: 0 mg

BAKED CINNAMON APPLES

Preparation Time: 10 min
Cooking Time: 25 min
Mode of Cooking: Baking
Servings: 4

Ingredients:
- 4 large apples, cored
- 2 Tbsp unsalted butter, melted
- 4 tsp cinnamon
- ¼ C. walnuts, chopped
- 2 Tbsp honey
- 1 tsp vanilla extract

Directions:
1. Preheat oven to 350°F (175°C)
2. Mix honey, melted butter, cinnamon, and vanilla
3. Spoon this mixture into the center of each apple and top with walnuts
4. Place in a baking dish and cover with foil
5. Bake until apples are tender

Tips:
- Serve with a dollop of Greek yogurt for added protein
- Cinnamon and walnuts provide anti-inflammatory benefits

Nutritional Values: Calories: 210, Fat: 9g, Carbs: 34g, Protein: 2g, Sugar: 28g, Sodium: 5 mg, Potassium: 195 mg, Cholesterol: 15 mg

GRILLED PEACHES WITH HONEY

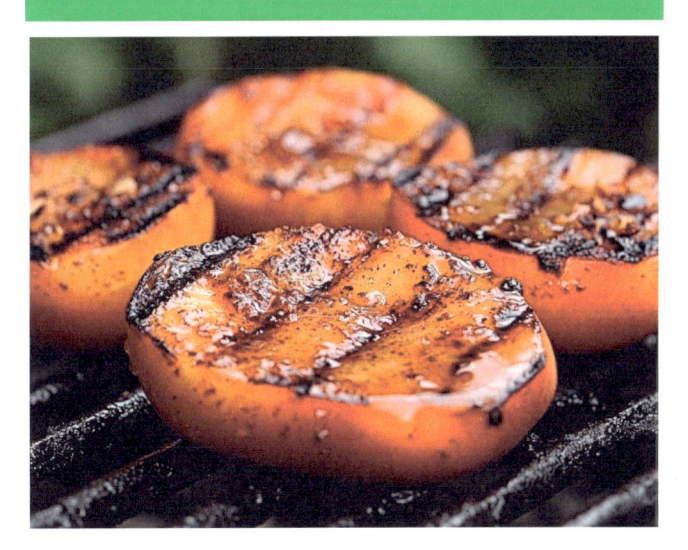

Preparation Time: 5 min
Cooking Time: 10 min
Mode of Cooking: Grilling
Servings: 4

Ingredients:
- 4 peaches, halved and pitted

- 2 Tbsp honey
- 1 tsp cinnamon
- coconut oil for grilling

Directions:

1. Preheat the grill to medium-high, brush peach halves with a light coat of coconut oil
2. Grill cut-side down until charred, about 5 min
3. Flip, drizzle with honey and sprinkle cinnamon, grill 5 more min.

Tips:

- Serve with a sprinkle of crushed almonds for extra crunch and nutrition
- Peaches are high in antioxidants which are anti-inflammatory

Nutritional Values: Calories: 120, Fat: 1g, Carbs: 29g, Protein: 2g, Sugar: 26g, Sodium: 0 mg, Potassium: 400 mg, Cholesterol: 0 mg

STRAWBERRY BASIL SALAD

Preparation Time: 10 min
Cooking Time: none
Mode of Cooking: Mixing
Servings: 4
Ingredients:

- 1 pt. strawberries, hulled and quartered
- 1 C. fresh basil leaves, loosely chopped
- 2 Tbsp balsamic vinegar
- 1 Tbsp extra virgin olive oil
- 1 tsp honey
- 1/4 C. sliced almonds

Directions:

1. In a bowl, combine strawberries and basil
2. Whisk together balsamic vinegar, olive oil, and honey to create a dressing
3. Drizzle over the strawberries and basil, and toss to coat
4. Top with sliced almonds

Tips:

- Salad can be chilled before serving for enhanced flavors
- The combination of strawberry and basil offers powerful phytonutrients and anti-inflammatory properties

Nutritional Values: Calories: 130, Fat: 7g, Carbs: 15g, Protein: 2g, Sugar: 10g, Sodium: 3 mg, Potassium: 170 mg, Cholesterol: 0 mg

BLUEBERRY CHIA PUDDING

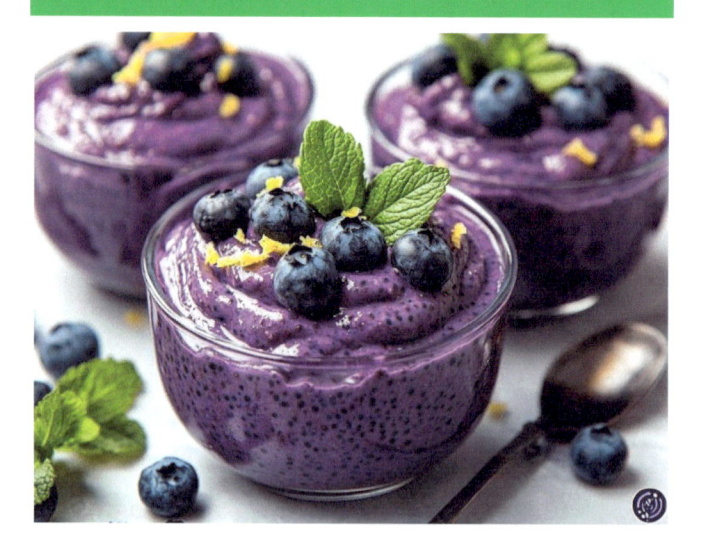

Preparation Time: 10 min
Cooking Time: 0 min (plus 4 hrs chilling)
Mode of Cooking: Mixing
Servings: 4

Ingredients:
- 2 C. coconut milk
- 1/2 C. chia seeds
- 1 C. blueberries, fresh or frozen
- 1 Tbsp honey
- 1 tsp vanilla extract
- zest of 1 lemon

Directions:
1. Mix chia seeds and coconut milk in a bowl, stir in honey, vanilla, and lemon zest
2. Cover and refrigerate for at least 4 hrs or overnight
3. Stir in fresh blueberries before serving

Tips:
- Add a sprinkle of ground flax seeds for an Omega-3 boost
- Blueberries are high in antioxidants, which combat inflammation

Nutritional Values: Calories: 200, Fat: 12g, Carbs: 20g, Protein: 4g, Sugar: 8g, Sodium: 30 mg, Potassium: 125 mg, Cholesterol: 0 mg

CARROT AND WALNUT MUFFINS

Preparation Time: 20 min
Cooking Time: 25 min
Mode of Cooking: Baking
Servings: 12

Ingredients:
- 1½ C. whole wheat flour
- ¾ C. brown sugar
- 1 tsp baking powder
- ½ tsp baking soda
- ¼ tsp salt
- 1 tsp cinnamon
- 2 C. shredded carrots
- ¾ C. unsweetened applesauce
- 2 eggs
- ¼ C. olive oil
- ½ C. walnuts, chopped

Directions:
1. Preheat oven to 375°F (190°C)
2. In a large bowl, sift together flour, baking powder, baking soda, salt, and cinnamon
3. In another bowl, mix eggs, applesauce, and olive oil
4. Stir in brown sugar until well combined
5. Add shredded carrots and walnuts to wet mixture
6. Combine wet and dry ingredients until just mixed
7. Spoon batter into greased muffin cups
8. Bake for 25 min or until a toothpick inserted comes out clean

Tips:
- Shredding carrots finely can help distribute moisture evenly
- Cinnamon not only adds flavor but also provides anti-inflammatory benefits
- Substitute walnuts with almonds for a change in texture and extra anti-inflammatory effects

Nutritional Values: Calories: 165, Fat: 9g, Carbs: 20g, Protein: 3g, Sugar: 11g, Sodium: 180 mg, Potassium: 120 mg, Cholesterol: 35 mg

Oatmeal Raisin Cookies

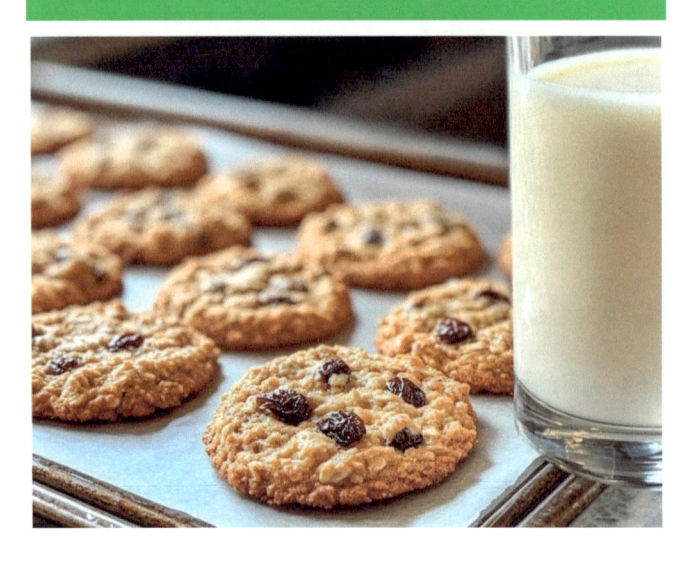

Preparation Time: 15 min
Cooking Time: 10 min
Mode of Cooking: Baking
Servings: 24
Ingredients:

- 1 C. rolled oats
- ¾ C. whole wheat flour
- ½ C. raisins
- 1 tsp baking soda
- ½ tsp cinnamon
- ¼ tsp salt
- ½ C. unsweetened applesauce
- ¼ C. coconut oil, melted
- ½ C. agave syrup
- 1 egg
- 1 tsp vanilla extract

Directions:

1. Preheat oven to 350°F (175°C)
2. In a bowl, mix oats, flour, baking soda, cinnamon, and salt
3. In another bowl, combine applesauce, coconut oil, agave syrup, egg, and vanilla extract
4. Mix wet ingredients into dry until just combined
5. Stir in raisins
6. Drop tablespoons of dough onto a lined baking sheet
7. Flatten slightly
8. Bake for 10 min or until edges are golden brown

Tips:

- Soaking raisins in warm water before adding can enhance their flavor and texture
- Cinnamon can be increased for added health benefits and richer flavor
- Agave syrup is a healthier alternative to refined sugars and helps keep inflammation at bay

Nutritional Values: Calories: 110, Fat: 4g, Carbs: 18g, Protein: 2g, Sugar: 8g, Sodium: 80 mg, Potassium: 75 mg, Cholesterol: 10 mg

Lemon Poppy Seed Scones

Preparation Time: 20 min
Cooking Time: 25 min
Mode of Cooking: Baking
Servings: 12
Ingredients:

- 2 C. all-purpose flour
- ½ C. sugar
- 1 Tbsp baking powder
- ¼ tsp salt
- 1 Tbsp poppy seeds
- 1 Tbsp lemon zest
- ¼ C. unsalted butter, cold and cubed
- 1 egg

- ¾ C. heavy cream
- ¼ tsp vanilla extract

Directions:

1. Preheat oven to 400°F (200°C)
2. In a large bowl, combine flour, sugar, baking powder, salt, poppy seeds, and lemon zest
3. Add cubed butter and mix until the mixture resembles coarse crumbs
4. In a separate bowl, whisk together egg, heavy cream, and vanilla extract
5. Gradly add wet ingredients to dry, mixing until dough forms
6. Turn dough onto a floured surface and shape into a round disc
7. Cut into wedges
8. Place on a baking sheet and bake for 25 min or until golden brown

Tips:

- Using cold butter in the scone dough will help achieve a flaky texture
- Lemon zest not only enhances the flavor but contributes vitamin C, aiding in anti-inflammatory and immune-boosting efforts
- Poppy seeds are packed with antioxidants and fiber which enhance the nutritional profile

Nutritional Values: Calories: 155, Fat: 7g, Carbs: 22g, Protein: 3g, Sugar: 7g, Sodium: 150 mg, Potassium: 60 mg, Cholesterol: 45 mg

CASHEW LIME DREAM BITES

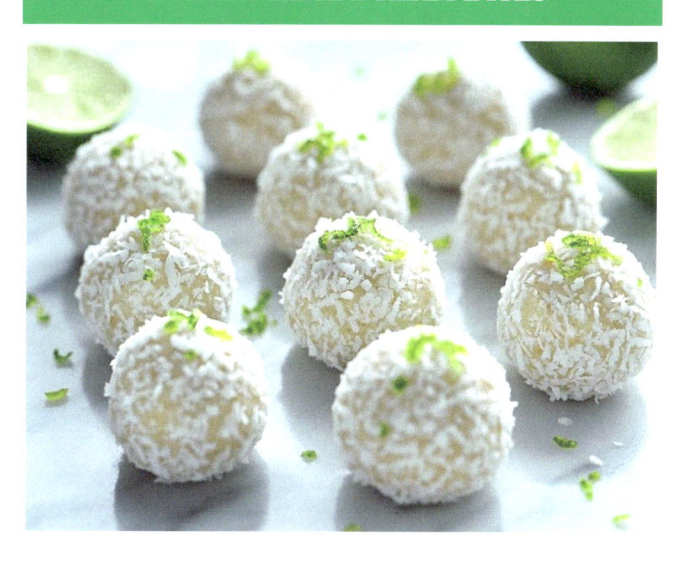

Preparation Time: 15 min.
Cooking Time: none
Mode of Cooking: No Cooking
Servings: 15

Ingredients:

- 1½ C. raw cashews
- 1 C. dates, pitted
- zest of 1 lime
- juice of 2 limes
- ¼ C. shredded coconut, unsweetened
- 1 Tbsp chia seeds
- pinch of sea salt

Directions:

1. Soak cashews in water for 4 hr., then drain
2. Blend dates, lime zest, lime juice, and salt in a food processor until smooth
3. Add softened cashews and pulse until mixture forms a sticky dough
4. Roll mixture into balls and coat with shredded coconut
5. Refrigerate for 2 hr. to set

Tips:

- Serve chilled for a refreshing treat
- Can be stored in an airtight container in the refrigerator for up to one week
- Zest and lime juice add a burst of flavor while acting as natural preservatives

Nutritional Values: Calories: 180, Fat: 9g, Carbs: 23g, Protein: 4g, Sugar: 15g, Sodium: 10 mg, Potassium: 210 mg, Cholesterol: 0 mg

AVOCADO CHOCOLATE MOUSSE

Preparation Time: 10 min.
Cooking Time: none
Mode of Cooking: No Cooking
Servings: 4

Ingredients:

- 2 ripe avocados
- ¼ C. raw cacao powder
- ¼ C. honey or maple syrup
- 1 tsp vanilla extract
- pinch of sea salt
- raspberries for garnish

Directions:

1. Blend avocados, cacao powder, honey, vanilla extract, and sea salt until smooth and creamy
2. Divide mousse among serving dishes
3. Garnish with raspberries
4. Chill in the refrigerator before serving

Tips:

- Opt for maple syrup if vegan
- Adding a pinch of cinnamon can enhance the flavor and add another layer of anti-inflammatory properties
- Raspberries not only add color but also provide additional antioxidants

Nutritional Values: Calories: 245, Fat: 15g, Carbs: 28g, Protein: 3g, Sugar: 17g, Sodium: 20 mg, Potassium: 487 mg, Cholesterol: 0 mg

Chapter 11: Beverages and Teas

There's something truly soothing about sipping on a warm cup of tea or refreshing beverage that nourishes your body and calms your mind. In this journey to transform our diet and manage inflammation, we often focus on solid meals, but let's not overlook the power of what we drink. Whether you start your day with a smoothie or unwind in the evening with a herbal tea, each sip is a step towards better health.

Beverages and teas, in the context of an anti-inflammatory lifestyle, are not just delightful additions; they are potent vehicles for vitamins, minerals, and antioxidants that fight inflammation and boost our immune system. Imagine harnessing the natural anti-inflammatory properties of ginger in a warm, invigorating ginger tea or capturing the antioxidants of berries in a chilled smoothie. These drinks do more than quench your thirst—they rejuvenate your body from the inside out.

However, navigating the world of beverages can be tricky. Commercial drinks often promise health benefits but are laden with sugars and artificial ingredients that can, contradictorily, trigger inflammation. Here, we take a different route. I'll introduce you to simple, homemade recipes that are not only easy to prepare but are assured to respect the principles of an anti-inflammatory diet. From the energizing kick of a green tea latte to the soothing embrace of a chamomile infusion, these beverages are designed to blend seamlessly into your daily routine, offering relaxation and health benefits without any hidden setbacks.

Furthermore, as we explore these recipes, remember that consistency is key. Integrating these drinks into your daily regimen can significantly enhance your digestive health, reduce stress levels, and ultimately, contribute to a sustained lifestyle shift toward better health. So, let's raise our glasses (or mugs!) to a deliciously wholesome chapter of our dietary journey. Here's to making every sip count towards a healthier, vibrant you!

Turmeric Ginger Tea

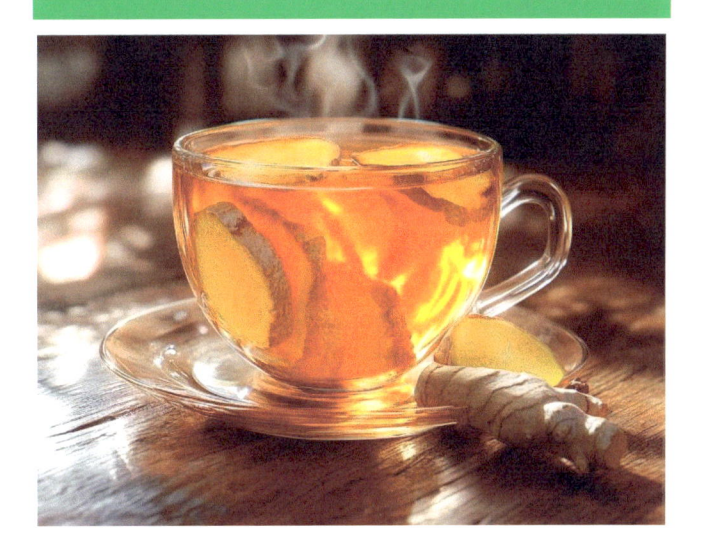

Preparation Time: 5 min
Cooking Time: 10 min
Mode of Cooking: Simmering
Servings: 2
Ingredients:
- 1 inch fresh turmeric root, thinly sliced

- 1 inch fresh ginger root, thinly sliced
- 4 cups water
- 1 Tbsp honey
- Juice of 1/2 lemon

Directions:

1. Combine turmeric and ginger with water in a saucepan and bring to boil
2. Reduce heat and simmer for 10 min
3. Remove from heat, add lemon juice and honey, stir well, and strain into cups

Tips:

- Add a pinch of black pepper to enhance curcumin absorption
- Honey can be replaced with maple syrup for a different sweetness
- Enjoy this tea warm or chilled for refreshing twist

Nutritional Values: Calories: 10, Fat: 0g, Carbs: 3g, Protein: 0g, Sugar: 2g, Sodium: 5 mg, Potassium: 20 mg, Cholesterol: 0 mg

CHAMOMILE AND LAVENDER TEA

Preparation Time: 3 min
Cooking Time: 5 min
Mode of Cooking: Steeping
Servings: 2
Ingredients:

- 2 Tbsp dried chamomile flowers
- 1 Tbsp dried lavender buds
- 3 cups boiling water
- 1 tsp raw honey

Directions:

1. Place chamomile and lavender in a teapot
2. Pour boiling water over the herbs and steep for 5 min
3. Strain into cups and stir in honey

Tips:

- Serve this tea before bedtime to promote relaxation and improve sleep quality
- A slice of lemon can be added for a citrusy twist or to enhance flavor

Nutritional Values: Calories: 5, Fat: 0g, Carbs: 1g, Protein: 0g, Sugar: 1g, Sodium: 0 mg, Potassium: 10 mg, Cholesterol: 0 mg

PEPPERMINT AND LICORICE ROOT TEA

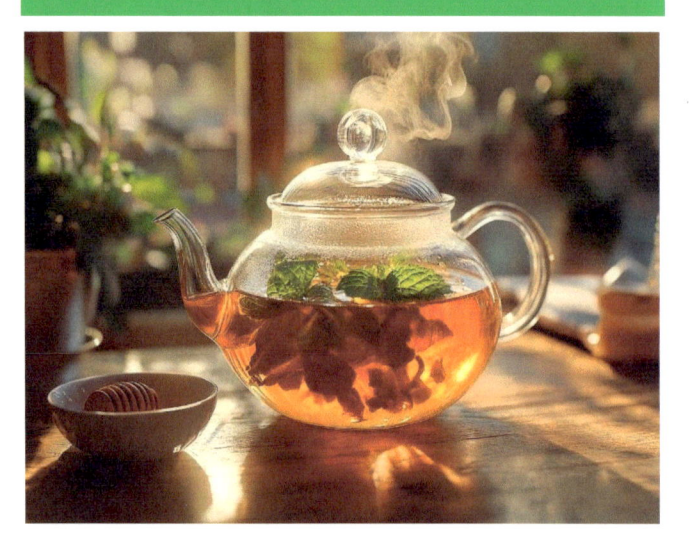

Preparation Time: 5 min
Cooking Time: 10 min
Mode of Cooking: Simmering
Servings: 2
Ingredients:

- 2 Tbsp dried peppermint leaves
- 1 Tbsp licorice root, chopped
- 4 cups water

Directions:

1. Combine peppermint leaves and licorice root in a pot with water and bring to a boil
2. Lower heat and simmer for 10 min

3. Strain and serve

Tips:

• This tea can be sweetened with honey or enjoyed unsweetened for a pure herbal flavor

• Peppermint is excellent for digestion and licorice root for soothing inflammation

Nutritional Values: Calories: 0, Fat: 0g, Carbs: 0g, Protein: 0g, Sugar: 0g, Sodium: 0 mg, Potassium: 5 mg, Cholesterol: 0 mg

HIBISCUS AND ROSEHIP TEA

Preparation Time: 4 min
Cooking Time: 6 min
Mode of Cooking: Boiling
Servings: 2
Ingredients:

- 2 Tbsp dried hibiscus flowers
- 1 Tbsp dried rosehips
- 3 cups boiling water
- 1 Tbsp honey

Directions:

1. Put hibiscus and rosehips into a pot
2. Pour boiling water over and let it steep for 6 min
3. Strain into cups and sweeten with honey as desired

Tips:

• A dash of cinnamon can be added for extra flavor and to boost anti-inflammatory properties

• Serve iced for a refreshing summer drink

• Hibiscus is known for its high vitamin C content and anti-inflammatory benefits

Nutritional Values: Calories: 5, Fat: 0g, Carbs: 2g, Protein: 0g, Sugar: 1g, Sodium: 0 mg, Potassium: 15 mg, Cholesterol: 0 mg

LEMON BALM AND GINGER INFUSION

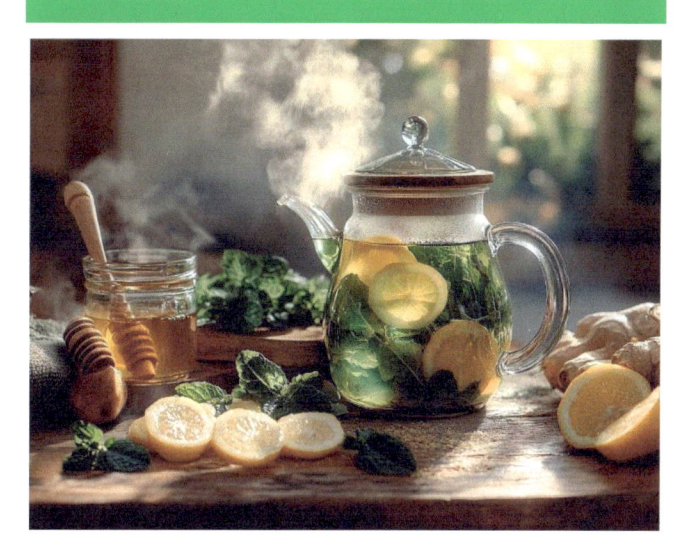

Preparation Time: 5 min
Cooking Time: 10 min
Mode of Cooking: Infusing
Servings: 2
Ingredients:

- 2 Tbsp lemon balm leaves, fresh
- 1 inch ginger root, minced
- 4 cups water
- Optional: 1 tsp honey

Directions:

1. Combine lemon balm and ginger in a pot with water and bring to a boil
2. Remove from heat and let sit, covered, for 10 min
3. Strain and serve, sweetening with honey if desired

Tips:

• Lemon balm can be grown in home gardens for freshness and ease

- This infusion can also be enjoyed cold, stored in the refrigerator for up to 24 hours

Nutritional Values: Calories: 2, Fat: 0g, Carbs: 1g, Protein: 0g, Sugar: 0g, Sodium: 0 mg, Potassium: 10 mg, Cholesterol: 0 mg

GOLDEN MILK SMOOTHIE

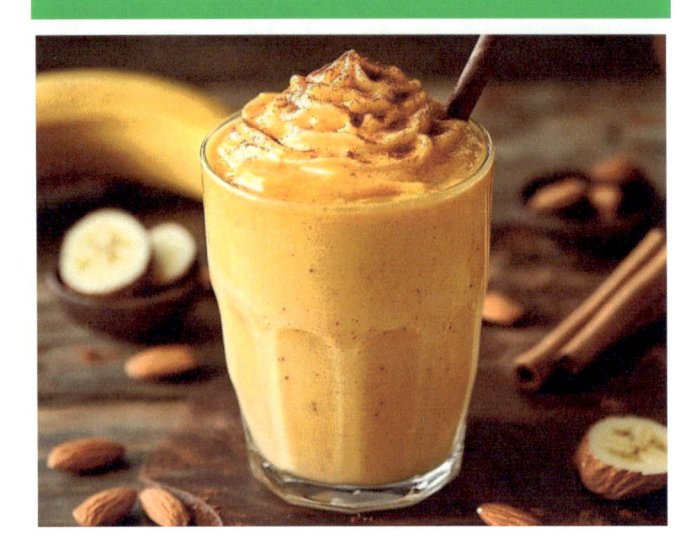

Preparation Time: 5 min.
Cooking Time: none
Mode of Cooking: Blending
Servings: 2
Ingredients:
- 1 ½ cups coconut milk
- 1 Tbsp turmeric paste
- 1 banana
- ½ tsp cinnamon
- 1 Tbsp almond butter
- 1 tsp vanilla extract
- Ice cubes as needed

Directions:
1. Blend coconut milk, turmeric paste, banana, cinnamon, almond butter, and vanilla extract together in a blender
2. Add ice cubes to reach preferred thickness and blend until creamy and smooth

Tips:
- Utilize freshly made turmeric paste for the best flavor and health benefits
- Incorporate a pinch of black pepper to enhance curcumin absorption from turmeric
- Ideal for an anti-inflammatory boost any time of the day

Nutritional Values: Calories: 310, Fat: 18g, Carbs: 29g, Protein: 4g, Sugar: 15g, Sodium: 40 mg, Potassium: 550 mg, Cholesterol: 0 mg

GREEN MATCHA SMOOTHIE

Preparation Time: 5 min.
Cooking Time: none
Mode of Cooking: Blending
Servings: 2
Ingredients:
- 1 cup unsweetened almond milk
- 1 tsp matcha green tea powder
- 1 banana, sliced
- ½ avocado, peeled and pitted
- 1 Tbsp honey
- Ice cubes as needed

Directions:
1. Combine almond milk, matcha powder, banana, avocado, and honey in a blender
2. Add ice cubes to desired consistency and blend until smooth

Tips:
- Opt for organic matcha to enhance the smoothie's anti-inflammatory properties

- Add a sprinkle of chia seeds for extra fiber and omega-3 fatty acids
- Enjoy this smoothie as a rejuvenating morning beverage

Nutritional Values: Calories: 245, Fat: 11g, Carbs: 35g, Protein: 3g, Sugar: 20g, Sodium: 40 mg, Potassium: 487 mg, Cholesterol: 0 mg

BLUEBERRY SPINACH SMOOTHIE

Preparation Time: 5 min.
Cooking Time: none
Mode of Cooking: Blending
Servings: 2
Ingredients:
- 1 cup fresh spinach
- 1 cup blueberries, frozen
- 1 banana
- 1 Tbsp flaxseeds
- 1 cup Greek yogurt, unsweetened
- ½ cup almond milk
- 1 tsp honey

Directions:
1. Place spinach, blueberries, banana, flaxseeds, Greek yogurt, almond milk, and honey in a blender
2. Blend until mixture is smooth and evenly mixed

Tips:
- Add a scoop of protein powder for an extra protein kick
- Replace honey with maple syrup for a vegan option
- Packed with antioxidants and omega-3s, this smoothie is perfect for an energy-boosting snack

Nutritional Values: Calories: 280, Fat: 7g, Carbs: 44g, Protein: 14g, Sugar: 28g, Sodium: 80 mg, Potassium: 470 mg, Cholesterol: 10 mg

GINGER BEET SMOOTHIE

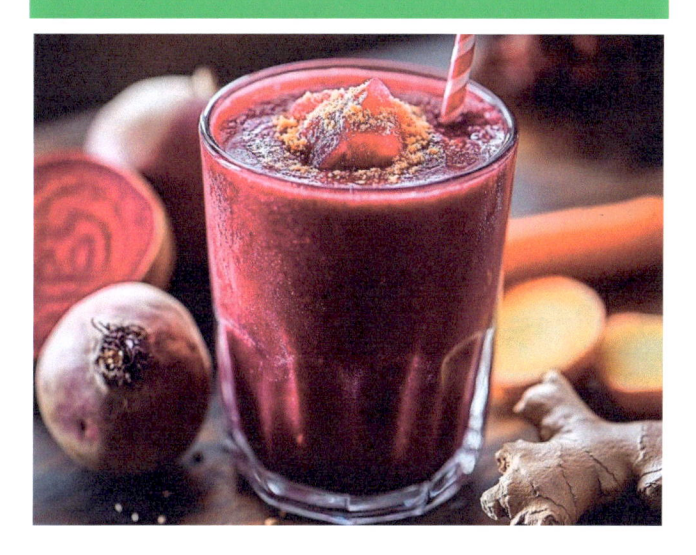

Preparation Time: 7 min.
Cooking Time: none
Mode of Cooking: Blending
Servings: 2
Ingredients:
- 1 medium beet, peeled and diced
- 1 apple, cored and sliced
- ½ inch piece ginger, peeled
- 1 carrot, peeled and chopped
- 1 cup water
- Juice of 1 lemon
- Ice cubes as needed

Directions:
1. Combine beet, apple, ginger, carrot, water, and lemon juice in a blender
2. Blend until smooth, adding ice to achieve desired thickness

Tips:

- Incorporate a tablespoon of hemp seeds for added protein and a nutty flavor
- Drink this vibrant smoothie to kickstart your metabolism and soothe inflammation

Nutritional Values: Calories: 180, Fat: 1g, Carbs: 43g, Protein: 3g, Sugar: 30g, Sodium: 90 mg, Potassium: 690 mg, Cholesterol: 0 mg

PINEAPPLE KALE SMOOTHIE

Preparation Time: 5 min.
Cooking Time: none
Mode of Cooking: Blending
Servings: 2

Ingredients:

- 1 cup chopped kale, stems removed
- 1 cup pineapple, cubed
- 1 banana
- 1/2 avocado
- 1 cup coconut water
- 1 Tbsp lemon juice
- Ice cubes as needed

Directions:

1. Put kale, pineapple, banana, avocado, coconut water, and lemon juice in a blender
2. Process until the texture is creamy and smooth

Tips:

- Sprinkle in some ground ginger for additional anti-inflammatory benefits
- Consider freezing the banana and pineapple beforehand for a thicker smoothie
- A powerful drink for reducing inflammation and boosting hydration

Nutritional Values: Calories: 215, Fat: 8g, Carbs: 37g, Protein: 3g, Sugar: 20g, Sodium: 70 mg, Potassium: 750 mg, Cholesterol: 0 mg

Chapter 12: Conclusion

As we draw to a close in this journey through the super easy anti-inflammatory diet, it's important to take a moment to reflect on the strides we've taken together. Launching into a new dietary habit is never a small feat, especially when it involves rethinking how you choose, prepare, and enjoy food. Yet, you've embarked on this path not just to change your diet, but to transform your life.

Understanding inflammation and its impact on your well-being was our starting point. We explored how this natural process, while vital, can become a persistent issue leading to various health challenges if not managed properly. By diving into what triggers inflammation and identifying symptoms that many struggle with daily, it established a fundamental reason for considering dietary changes seriously.

As you progressed through the book, we laid out the anti-inflammatory foods and the unwanted ones, stirring your kitchen's transformation. These lists were not just guides but invitations to experiment with flavors while nurturing your body. Through detailed discussions about essential nutrients like Omega-3 fatty acids, antioxidants, and phytochemicals, the goal was to arm you with knowledge to make informed food choices.

Every recipe introduced was crafted to ease your routine, not complicate it. Breakfasts designed to invigorate, lunches that could be splendid yet simple, dinners that unite and heal, and snacks and treats to satisfy without the guilt. Each meal was a building block towards a healthier you. But it wasn't just about the meals; it was about setting a table where well-being was always the honored guest.

Through the 30-day meal plan, the aim was to help you visualize this journey, making it tangible and approachable. Each day suggested a path, yet each was open to your tweaks and twists, encouraging you to embrace flexibility and creativity in your diet. This plan wasn't merely a schedule; it was a starting line from where life's race towards better health begins anew each day.

In closing this chapter, let's consider not just what you will take away, but how you will move forward. Adopting an anti-inflammatory diet is not merely a phase but a sustained lifestyle choice. It's about more than alleviating symptoms; it's about setting a new standard for your life quality. The changes you've started to implement should grow with you, adaptable and enduring.

Remember, the transition to an anti-inflammatory diet doesn't mean conforming to a rigid set of rules but rather understanding what works best for your body. Nutrition is deeply personal and what works for one person might not suit another. This is about listening to your body, recognizing its signals and responding with love and care through your dietary choices.

Moreover, stress, a pervasive ailment in our fast-paced world, has a pronounced effect on inflammation. An integral part of your journey is finding balance and serenity not just on your plate but in your mind. Techniques that promote relaxation and stress reduction, such as mindfulness, yoga, or simple daily gratitude, can amplify the benefits of the dietary changes you are making.

As this book ends, think of it not as the conclusion of an experiment, but the foundation of your lifestyle. Continue exploring, learning, and adapting. Keep your meals colorful, your body nourished, and your mind at ease. Know that with every bite of a well-thought-out meal, you're taking a step towards a more vibrant, healthier life.

If there's one thing to carry with you, let it be the understanding that your journey to health is an ever-evolving process. Setbacks may occur, and that's perfectly normal. The key is to remain committed, be gentle with yourself, and focus on progression, not perfection.

Together, we've looked at diets not just as a part of medical advice but as a piece of a holistic approach to wellness. The road to diminishing inflammation and enhancing your life through diet is ongoing; your engagement and willingness to adapt are what will sustain these changes. Therefore, keep your curiosity alive, continue to seek knowledge and uphold the belief that within you lies the power to influence your health profoundly.

Thank you for sharing this part of your health journey with me. Until we meet on these pages again, may your meals be tasty, your spirits high, and your body free from the burden of inflammation. Here's to your health — refreshed, renewed, and ever-inspiring.

30 DAYS MEAL PLAN

Embarking on a new dietary plan often brings a mix of excitement and apprehension. How do we transform the aspirational vision of healthier eating into daily reality? The "30 Days Meal Plan" is crafted to act as your navigational tool through the invigorating world of the anti-inflammatory diet, helping to dissolve the barriers between you and your health objectives.

Imagine a bridge spanning the gap between understanding the benefits of an anti-inflammatory lifestyle and actualizing daily habits that reflect this knowledge. This meal plan is designed to be that bridge. Each day's menu is more than just a collection of recipes—it's a day in your new life, one where your dietary choices actively contribute to reducing inflammation, enhancing digestion, and bolstering your immune system.

The beauty of this 30-day guide lies in its simplicity and flexibility. No day is a carbon copy of another, ensuring that your meals remain exciting and diverse. This not only suits your palate but also addresses the common concern that a health-focused diet might lack in variety or flavor. From vibrant breakfast smoothies packed with antioxidants to soothing, spice-infused dinners that promise to be as comforting as they are healthful, every recipe is designed to be straightforward and quick to prepare—a perfect fit for your busy schedule.

Moreover, this plan isn't just about feeding the body but also about nurturing the soul. Stress reduction is woven into the fabric of this meal plan. Whether it's through enjoying a quiet moment with a warm, nutritious lunch or the satisfaction of preparing a colorful salad that looks as delightful as it tastes, every meal is an opportunity to step back and breathe a little easier.

As you progress through these 30 days, each meal will reinforce the connection between what you eat and how you feel. It's a journey of discovery, taste, and health—a true testament to how small, manageable changes can culminate in profound improvements in your quality of life. Let's embark on this promising journey together, one flavorful, nourishing meal at a time.

	breakfast	snack	lunch	snack	dinner
Day 01	Golden Turmeric Morning Elixir	Beetroot and Apple Juice	Kale and Quinoa Power Bowl	Almond Coconut Energy Balls	Herb-Marinated Grilled Salmon
Day 02	Blueberry Avocado Bliss Smoothie	Carrot Ginger Smoothie	Chickpea and Avocado Garden Salad	Turmeric Cashew Bites	Lemon Garlic Chicken Breasts
Day 03	Green Detox Power Smoothie	Green Apple Kale Juice	Turkey and Spinach Sandwich	Date and Walnut Bars	Spiced Tofu Stir-Fry
Day 04	Spiced Berry Metabolism Booster	Berry Antioxidant Smoothie	Roasted Beet and Arugula Salad	Chia Seed Energy Bites	Ginger-Lime Shrimp
Day 05	Pineapple Ginger Immune Booster	Pineapple Turmeric Juice	Mediterranean Lentil Bowl	Pumpkin Spice Protein Balls	Balsamic Glazed Pork Chops
Day 06	Turmeric Ginger Chia Pudding	Almond Coconut Energy Balls	Coconut Curry Soup	Beetroot and Apple Juice	Roasted Cauliflower Steaks with Turmeric and Garlic
Day 07	Omega Booster Smoothie Bowl	Turmeric Cashew Bites	Grilled Chicken Wrap	Carrot Ginger Smoothie	Zucchini Noodles with Avocado Pesto
Day 08	Savory Quinoa Breakfast Bowl	Date and Walnut Bars	Hummus and Veggie Sandwich	Green Apple Kale Juice	Cauliflower Mac and Cheese
Day 09	Berry Antioxidant Oatmeal	Chia Seed Energy Bites	Avocado Chickpea Wrap	Berry Antioxidant Smoothie	Lentil Bolognese
Day 10	Sweet Potato & Kale Hash	Pumpkin Spice Protein Balls	Turkey and Spinach Sandwich	Pineapple Turmeric Juice	Chicken and Veggie Casserole

	breakfast	snack	lunch	snack	dinner
Day 11	Turmeric Ginger Chia Pudding	Pineapple Turmeric Juice	Spinach and Strawberry Crisp Salad	Carrot Ginger Smoothie	Spiced Tofu Stir-Fry
Day 12	Spiced Berry Metabolism Booster	Turmeric Cashew Bites	Mediterranean Lentil Bowl	Almond Coconut Energy Balls	Lemon Garlic Chicken Breasts
Day 13	Blueberry Avocado Bliss Smoothie	Pumpkin Spice Protein Balls	Hummus and Veggie Sandwich	Green Apple Kale Juice	Cauliflower Mac and Cheese
Day 14	Savory Quinoa Breakfast Bowl	Berry Antioxidant Smoothie	Grilled Chicken Wrap	Pineapple Turmeric Juice	Roasted Cauliflower Steaks with Turmeric and Garlic
Day 15	Omega Booster Smoothie Bowl	Date and Walnut Bars	Spinach and Strawberry Crisp Salad	Date and Walnut Bars	Balsamic Glazed Pork Chops
Day 16	Golden Turmeric Morning Elixir	Beetroot and Apple Juice	Chickpea and Avocado Garden Salad	Beetroot and Apple Juice	Ginger-Lime Shrimp
Day 17	Green Detox Power Smoothie	Green Apple Kale Juice	Roasted Beet and Arugula Salad	Pumpkin Spice Protein Balls	Chicken and Veggie Casserole
Day 18	Sweet Potato & Kale Hash	Almond Coconut Energy Balls	Avocado Chickpea Wrap	Chia Seed Energy Bites	Lentil Bolognese
Day 19	Pineapple Ginger Immune Booster	Carrot Ginger Smoothie	Coconut Curry Soup	Turmeric Cashew Bites	Herb-Marinated Grilled Salmon
Day 20	Berry Antioxidant Oatmeal	Chia Seed Energy Bites	Kale and Quinoa Power Bowl	Berry Antioxidant Smoothie	Zucchini Noodles with Avocado Pesto

	breakfast	snack	lunch	snack	dinner
Day 21	Blueberry Avocado Bliss Smoothie	Berry Antioxidant Smoothie	Roasted Beet and Arugula Salad	Carrot Ginger Smoothie	Ginger-Lime Shrimp
Day 22	Spiced Berry Metabolism Booster	Pineapple Turmeric Juice	Avocado Chickpea Wrap	Almond Coconut Energy Balls	Roasted Cauliflower Steaks with Turmeric and Garlic
Day 23	Berry Antioxidant Oatmeal	Beetroot and Apple Juice	Grilled Chicken Wrap	Date and Walnut Bars	Zucchini Noodles with Avocado Pesto
Day 24	Savory Quinoa Breakfast Bowl	Green Apple Kale Juice	Turkey and Spinach Sandwich	Green Apple Kale Juice	Spiced Tofu Stir-Fry
Day 25	Golden Turmeric Morning Elixir	Almond Coconut Energy Balls	Coconut Curry Soup	Pumpkin Spice Protein Balls	Lentil Bolognese
Day 26	Sweet Potato & Kale Hash	Pumpkin Spice Protein Balls	Hummus and Veggie Sandwich	Pineapple Turmeric Juice	Chicken and Veggie Casserole
Day 27	Green Detox Power Smoothie	Turmeric Cashew Bites	Mediterranean Lentil Bowl	Chia Seed Energy Bites	Lemon Garlic Chicken Breasts
Day 28	Omega Booster Smoothie Bowl	Date and Walnut Bars	Kale and Quinoa Power Bowl	Turmeric Cashew Bites	Herb-Marinated Grilled Salmon
Day 29	Pineapple Ginger Immune Booster	Carrot Ginger Smoothie	Spinach and Strawberry Crisp Salad	Beetroot and Apple Juice	Balsamic Glazed Pork Chops
Day 30	Turmeric Ginger Chia Pudding	Chia Seed Energy Bites	Chickpea and Avocado Garden Salad	Berry Antioxidant Smoothie	Cauliflower Mac and Cheese

Made in United States
Troutdale, OR
03/31/2025